Advanced Electrosurgery

Arash Taheri • Kasra Taheri • Bahram Hejrani
Zoubin Alikhani

Advanced Electrosurgery

Basics, Principles, and Applications

Springer

Arash Taheri
Jencare Senior Medical Center
Atlanta, GA, USA

Kasra Taheri
Atlanta International School
Atlanta, GA, USA

Bahram Hejrani
Stereotactic and Functional Neurosurgery
Philadelphia, PA, USA

Zoubin Alikhani
Atlanta Heart Specialists, LLC
Atlanta, GA, USA

ISBN 978-3-032-28341-2 ISBN 978-3-032-28342-9 (eBook)
https://doi.org/10.1007/978-3-032-28342-9

This Springer imprint is published by the registered company Springer Nature Switzerland AG
The registered company address is: Gewerbestrasse 11, 6330 Cham, Switzerland

Preface

The development of modern electrosurgery emerged from a collaboration between engineers and surgeons. However, miscommunication between these disciplines has led to inconsistencies in terminology and ambiguity in the proper use of key concepts. This lack of clarity has posed significant challenges to the standardization of electrosurgical methods, the effective teaching and learning of the subject, and the accurate performance and reporting of clinical studies.

Dr. Arash Taheri, a dermatologic surgeon with a strong foundation in the physics of electricity, encountered similar challenges early in his career in attempting to understand and confidently utilize electrosurgery. Driven by these difficulties, he devoted himself to the systematic study of the field and established collaborations with engineers experienced in the design and manufacture of electrosurgical devices. After two decades of research, he has authored the first comprehensive book on electrosurgery written by an individual with deep expertise in both its physical principles and clinical practice.

As the most scientifically rigorous publication in this field to date, Dr. Taheri's book serves as a bridge between engineering and medicine. It provides surgeons and engineers with a clearer understanding of the fundamental principles and clinical applications of electrosurgery. Furthermore, by standardizing terminology, the work facilitates more effective communication, teaching, and research collaboration within the electrosurgical community.

Atlanta, GA, USA

Arash Taheri
Kasra Taheri

Acknowledgments

To my parents and teachers, Esmat and Iraj, who taught me how to think, study, work hard, and grow.

To my friend and teacher, Dr. Kamran Baligh, for his support and his time teaching me dermatology.

To Dr. Steven Feldman, who supported me to start a new chapter in my life in the United States.

To my partner in life and love, Parisa.

And special thanks to Kasra Taheri for English language editing of this book.

Contents

About the Authors

Arash Taheri is a Lead Physician, working as a geriatrician and dermatologist at Jencare Senior Medical Center. He completed his medical school, internship, and dermatology residency at Tehran University of Medical Science. He joined the Center for Dermatology Research at Wake Forest University in 2012 and completed his internal medicine residency at Wake Forest Department of Internal Medicine in 2017.

His chief clinical and research interests are electrosurgery and effects of high-frequency electrical currents on biological tissues. He has published multiple scientific articles in this field including two Continuing Medical Education articles in the *Journal of the American Academy of Dermatology*. He has been co-director for Electrosurgery and Cryosurgery Workshop at American Academy of Dermatology Annual Meeting 2017 and 2018.

Bahram Hejrani is a board-certified neurosurgeon trained in Iran. He completed a fellowship in Stereotactic and Functional Neurosurgery from 2015 to 2017. Dr. Hejrani has extensive experience in inserting deep brain stimulators for the treatment of various neurological conditions.

Zoubin Alikhani is the Director of Clinical Cardiac Electrophysiology Services and Arrhythmia Clinics at Atlanta Heart Specialists. He received his medical degree from Tehran University of Medical Sciences and completed advanced training in internal medicine, cardiology, and cardiac electrophysiology at Columbia University, Tufts University, and Harvard Medical School's Brigham and Women's Hospital.

Dr. Alikhani has authored numerous scientific publications and has presented his research at national and international meetings, including those of the Heart Rhythm Society. His academic interests include the biophysics of catheter ablation, with a particular focus on optimizing ablation strategies and advanced imaging modalities to enhance the precision of cardiac mapping and the treatment of complex arrhythmias. He is also recognized for his expertise in cardiac implantable electronic devices and directs one of the busiest device management clinics in the Atlanta metropolitan area.

Chapter 1
Definition of Terms and Introduction to Electrosurgical Methods and Modes

Abstract The development of modern-day electrosurgery was a collaboration between engineers and surgeons. However, it seems that some miscommunication between them resulted in confusion in the definition and proper use of terminology in this field. This confusion in terminology has caused major problems with the standardization of electrosurgical methods, the teaching and learning of electrosurgery, and performing and reporting clinical studies. Proper use of terminology makes understanding electrosurgery significantly easier.

This chapter provides a brief introduction to electrosurgical terms and methods. It is strongly recommended that readers study this chapter before starting the book to avoid confusion that may arise from misunderstandings of terms and definitions.

1.1 Definition of Terms in Electrosurgery

Electrosurgery: In electrosurgery, a high-frequency alternating electric current flows from an active electrode into tissue, generating heat and causing thermal tissue damage adjacent to the active electrode. An electrosurgical unit can be used either for burning (electrocoagulation) or cutting the tissue (electrosection) (Figs. 1.1 and 1.2).

- *Electrocoagulation* occurs when tissue is heated and undergoes thermal denaturation.
  Electrocoagulation can be performed in either spray method (fulguration) or contact method; however, the term electrocoagulation typically refers to coagulation in contact method.
  - In *fulguration*, the electrosurgical generator is activated first. The electrode then comes in contact with the tissue. When the activated electrode touches the tissue, sparks form. The current passes through the sparks and coagulates the tissue.
  - In *contact electrocoagulation* (traditionally called electrocoagulation), the electrode makes direct contact with the tissue before the generator is activated. The current passes directly from the electrode into the tissue without producing sparks.

A. Taheri et al., *Advanced Electrosurgery*,
https://doi.org/10.1007/978-3-032-28342-9_1

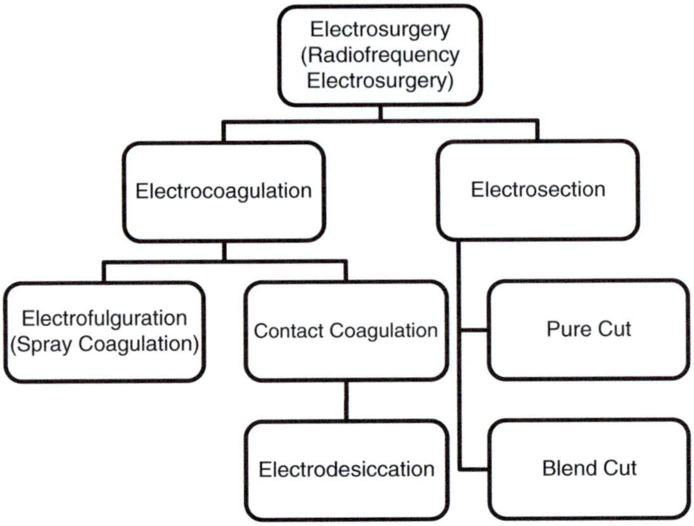

Fig. 1.1 Electrosurgery can be used to coagulate or cut. Electrocoagulation can be performed in spray (fulguration) mode or contact mode. Continuing contact coagulation up to tissue drying is called desiccation

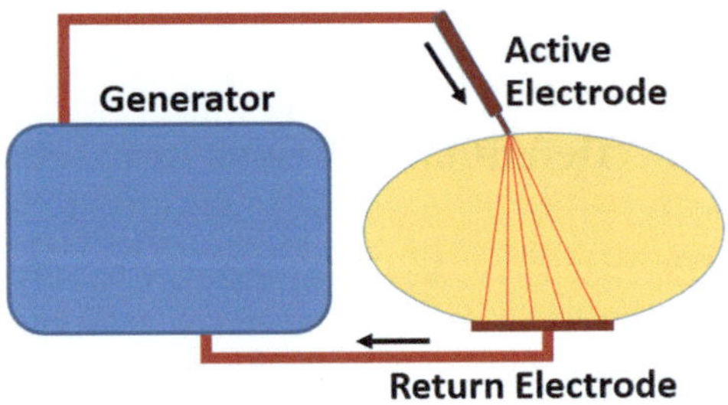

Fig. 1.2 An electrosurgical circuit. A high-frequency alternating current flows from an active electrode into the tissue, generating heat in the tissue adjacent to the active electrode

  - *Electrodesiccation.* With continuing current passage in contact coagulation, superficial coagulated tissue dries out, a process called desiccation. Once dried, this layer resists further current flow, often resulting in a popping sound and an onset of sparking (fulguration). Electrodesiccation is not an electrosurgical method or a distinctive final tissue effect. Rather, it is the final and deepest stage of contact coagulation that changes the current passage mode from contact to fulguration.

- *Electrosection* occurs when a very-high-density current passes through a tissue, causing a sudden increase in temperature. This leads to rapid, explosive vaporization of intracellular and extracellular water, which results in tissue fragmentation and cutting.
  - In pure cut, there is minimal coagulation on the incision walls.
  - In blend cut (a combination of cutting and coagulation), there is deeper coagulation on the incision walls, which provides improved hemostasis.

Radiofrequency Surgery: Electrosurgery is also known as radiofrequency surgery because the electrical currents used are in the radiofrequency range.

Electrocautery: Traditionally, the term electrocautery refers to hot wire cautery. In electrocautery, an electrical current passes through a metallic probe or wire, generating heat. This hot wire is then applied to tissue to cause coagulation. Importantly, no electrical current passes through the patient's body in electrocautery.

Diathermy: The term diathermy was originally used to describe the therapeutic (nonablative) heating effect of high-frequency electrical currents passing through the body. This term was later used to describe cutting tissue. To avoid confusion, the term diathermy should not be used when referring to cutting or coagulation.

Bipolar Electrosurgery: In bipolar electrosurgery, a bipolar forceps grasps the target tissue. The current passes from one tip of the forceps through the tissue to the other tip of the forceps. Thus, there are two active electrodes in contact with the target tissue for coagulation.

Monopolar Electrosurgery: There are one active and one dispersive (return) electrode. The return electrode may be connected to the patient (biterminal) or not (monoterminal).

Biterminal Electrosurgery: Both active and return electrodes are in contact with the patient's body.

Monoterminal Electrosurgery: The return electrode is not connected directly to the patient. Instead, it is grounded, and the earth acts as an indirect capacitive return electrode.

Electrosurgical Modes Versus Methods: In this book, the term *mode* refers to the generator's output setting selected via the device interface (e.g., fulguration, coagulation, or cut). Each mode determines the waveform of the current. The term *method* refers to the actual procedure performed. For example, a coagulation mode delivers an interrupted current, which can be used for any method, such as fulguration (spraying the current), contact coagulation, or cutting. This distinction between mode and method will be explored in greater detail throughout this book.

1.2 Introduction to Electrosurgical Methods

1.2.1 Electrocoagulation

Electrocoagulation can be performed using different methods. The most common methods for applying current in electrocoagulation are:

- *Fulguration*
  - *Fulguration using a fine-tip electrode (e.g., the tip of a needle or a knife-shaped electrode)*: In this method, the generator is activated first, and then the tip of the electrode is brought in contact with the tissue. Upon contact, sparks form. The electrode is moved by the surgeon along the tissue surface at a speed sufficient to cause coagulation. Although fulguration results in desiccation (drying) or even charring of the treated tissue, the term desiccation does not apply here.
  - *Fulguration using a large-interface electrode (e.g., the flat side of a knife or blade electrode)*: The procedure is performed similarly to fulguration using a fine-tip electrode. Compared with a fine-tip electrode, a large electrode functions like a larger brush, covering a larger surface area of tissue per unit of time.

- *Contact coagulation*
  - *Contact coagulation using a fine-tip electrode (e.g., the tip of a needle or a knife-shaped electrode)*: This method is generally used for superficial coagulation of small epidermal lesions. In this method, the generator is set to a very low power. The tip of the electrode is brought into contact with tissue. The generator is then activated, and the electrode is moved on the tissue surface at a speed sufficient to cause coagulation [1]. During this process, direct physical contact between the electrode and the tissue may be interrupted sometimes. If the electrode loses its contact with tissue, it may change the process to fulguration with spark formation.
  - *Contact coagulation using an electrode with a large tissue interface (e.g., a disk, a ball-shaped electrode, or the flat side of a knife or blade electrode)*: The large surface of the electrode is brought into complete contact with tissue. The generator is then activated, and the electrode is moved along the tissue surface at a speed sufficient to cause coagulation. This method is used for deep coagulation.
  - *Desiccation using an electrode with a large tissue interface (e.g., a disk, ball-shaped electrode, or the flat side of a knife or blade electrode).* This method is similar to contact coagulation using a large electrode, but the procedure continues after coagulation until desiccation is achieved. The large surface of the electrode is brought into complete contact with tissue. The generator is then activated. The electrode can stay in place until a popping sound is heard. For desiccation of larger surfaces, the electrode can be moved over the tissue at a speed slow enough to cause boiling of the water within the tissue. If an audible popping sound or sparking is noted, it indicates the final stage of desiccation and the start of fulguration. At this point, the generator can be deactivated, the tissue moistened again, and the sequence can be repeated to achieve deeper coagulation.

1.2.2 Electrosection

- *Pure cutting*: For a relatively clean incision with little hemostasis, a thin needle-shaped electrode and a continuous cutting current (cut mode) are used. Tissue cutting should be brisk, using the lowest possible power setting that still allows the surgeon to move quickly. A thick electrode cannot produce a pure, clean cut.
- *Blend cutting*: For better hemostasis, an interrupted current (blend or coagulation mode) is used with a needle-shaped or knife electrode. This method provides a thicker layer of coagulation along the incision walls.

1.3 Applications of Electrosurgical Methods

- Fulguration can provide superficial coagulation if a relatively low power is used. It can also cause deeper tissue damage if a relatively higher power is used and the activated electrode is kept over a confined area for a longer duration.
- Contact coagulation can provide superficial coagulation when a small-tip electrode is used with a relatively low power. In contrast, contact coagulation using a large-tip electrode requires relatively high power and results in deeper coagulation.

Superficial coagulation of a small non-bleeding area, such as a small seborrheic keratosis, is best performed using a fine-tip electrode (e.g., the tip of a needle or a knife) in the contact method. Electrofulguration can also provide superficial coagulation of small areas.

Superficial coagulation of a very large area can be performed using the fulguration method. Contact coagulation does not have a role here, because a fine-tip electrode in the contact method is too slow and time-consuming for a large area. Also, a large-tip electrode in the contact method cannot provide superficial coagulation. Using a large-tip electrode for fulguration can work like a large brush and speed up the process when treating very large surfaces. Another advantage of using a large-tip electrode for fulguration is the more homogenous coagulation and better hemostasis it provides compared to a fine-tip electrode.

Deep coagulation of a large area, such as coagulation after curettage of a basal cell carcinoma, is best performed using a large-tip electrode (e.g., a ball-shaped electrode or the flat side of a knife or blade electrode) in the contact method. Fulguration with a large-tip electrode can also achieve a deep coagulation when higher power is used and the activated electrode is held over a confined area for a relatively longer time. However, this approach is slower than contact coagulation and generates significantly more smoke.

Deep coagulation of a very small area, or selective targeting of deeper tissues with minimal epidermal damage, can be performed using a penetrating needle-shaped active electrode inserted into the tissue or skin before the generator is activated. Insulation of the proximal part of the active electrode can protect the epidermis.

1.4 Introduction to Electrosurgical Modes and Current Waveforms

The cutting mode of electrosurgical generators uses a continuous waveform. Other modes—including blend cut, coagulation, and fulguration—deliver intermittent currents (Fig. 1.3).

Electrosection requires a high-power current, but the voltage should be relatively low to prevent the formation of large sparks. The cutting mode with its continuous waveform allows the generator to deliver maximum power output at a relatively low voltage.

Electrofulguration, by contrast, often requires a relatively low power to produce a superficial coagulation and a higher voltage to produce larger sparks. Intermittent current modes (coagulation or fulguration) reduce the output power while maintaining the maximum voltage of the current and can therefore be used for superficial fulguration.

It is important to note that the name of an electrosurgical waveform or mode (e.g., cutting mode, coagulation mode, or fulguration mode) does not necessarily determine its final surgical effect on tissue. A continuous current delivered in cutting mode can produce a clean cut, a blend cut, or even coagulation (including fulguration and desiccation), depending on how the current is applied. Conversely, an interrupted current from coagulation or fulguration modes can result in blend cutting or coagulation but not a pure cut.

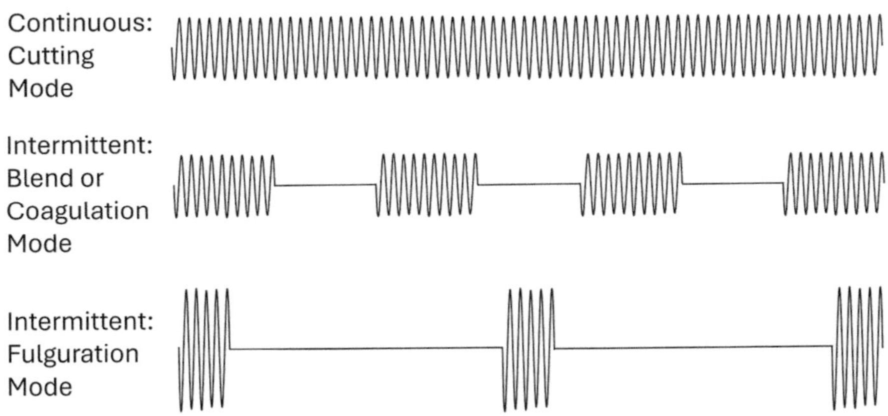

Fig. 1.3 Electrosurgical waveforms produced in different modes. An intermittent current waveform switches on and off thousands of times per second. As a result, it has a lower average power than a continuous current, since it is not active the entire time

Since the cutting mode of an electrosurgical unit can be used for all electrosurgical methods and also has the maximum power output of the device, this mode can be the default mode for performing most of the procedures. The most common reason a dermatologist may need to switch to fulguration mode is when sparks produced in cutting mode are not large enough for performing an efficient fulguration using a relatively small-tip electrode.

Reference

1. Taheri A, Mansoori P, Sandoval LF, Feldman SR, Pearce D, Williford PM. Electrosurgery: Part II. Technology, applications, and safety of electrosurgical devices. J Am Acad Dermatol. 2014;70(4):607.e1-12. https://doi.org/10.1016/j.jaad.2013.09.055. quiz 619–20. PubMed PMID: 24629362.

Chapter 2
Introduction to Electrosurgery

Abstract Electricity is used in surgery either as high-frequency electrosurgery (usually called electrosurgery) or as hot iron electrocautery (usually called electrocautery).

2.1 High-Frequency Electrosurgery

The term *electrosurgery* refers to the passage of a high-frequency alternating electrical current through tissue to achieve a specific surgical effect. As the current passes through the tissue in contact with the active electrode, the resistance of the tissue converts electrical energy into heat. *Electrocoagulation* occurs when tissue is heated and undergoes thermal denaturation. A sudden increase in tissue temperature above the boiling point causes rapid, explosive vaporization of the water content in the tissue adjacent to the electrode, leading to tissue fragmentation and *cutting*.

Unlike direct currents or low-frequency currents, high-frequency electrical currents do not cause cell depolarization or neuromuscular excitation.

2.2 Hot Wire Electrocautery

- In electrocautery, a metallic wire is heated by an electrical current, and the hot wire is then used to burn the tissue.
- In this method, no current passes through the tissue. This is in contrast with electrosurgery, where the current flows through the target. Because of this, electrocautery is safer for patients with implanted electronic devices.
- Hot wire electrocautery causes superficial tissue destruction unless it is kept on the tissue for a long time. Therefore, it is safer in inexperienced hands. Electrosurgery may be preferred over electrocautery when the treatment area is very large or very small.

A. Taheri et al., *Advanced Electrosurgery*,
https://doi.org/10.1007/978-3-032-28342-9_2

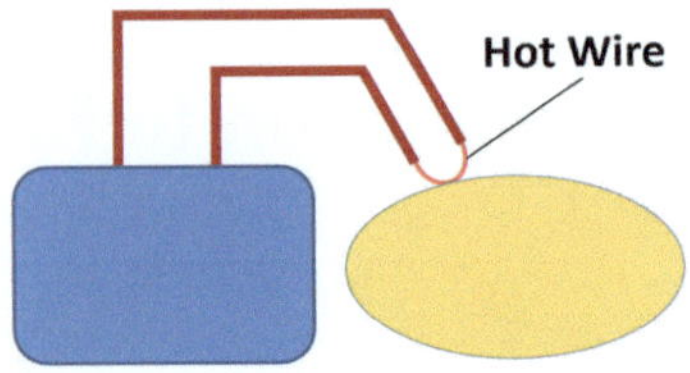

Fig. 2.1 An electrocautery circuit. An electric current heats the tip of the probe, which can then be used to heat superficial tissue layers. No current flows through the patient's body

Hot wire electrocautery was the first and simplest form of using electricity in surgery. In this method, a metallic wire is heated by a passing electrical current. Then the hot wire is used to burn the tissue (Fig. 2.1). Usually, a low-voltage direct current is used in electrocautery devices, because there is less chance for neuromuscular stimulation and electrical shock with these currents compared with higher voltages or low-frequency alternating currents. High-frequency currents are not used for electrocautery, because of the higher cost of producing these currents compared with direct currents and the higher risk of current leakage and unwanted burn associated with high frequency currents.

Low-voltage currents can be provided by batteries in handheld electrocautery devices or by a generator or adapter plugged into the wall. Larger devices that use wall-plugged generators usually have higher power as well as a dial to control the temperature of the wire. Handheld devices can be low temperature or high temperature, with no dial on the device to change the temperature.

In modern surgery, hot wire electrocautery is typically used when electrosurgical devices are not available or when the patient has a contraindication to alternating currents. Some implanted electronic devices in patients' bodies may be affected by high-frequency electrosurgical currents, making high-frequency electrosurgery unsuitable. Electrocautery is safe for these patients because no current passes through the patient's body during the procedure, eliminating concern for interference or damage to the implanted electronic devices.

A brief application of hot wire electrocautery causes superficial tissue coagulation. However, if the hot wire is kept in place for more than a few seconds, heat conduction may result in deeper coagulation.

Electrocautery is considered safer than electrosurgery because (a) the potential depth of tissue damage is less with electrocautery than with electrosurgery, (b) electrocautery does not interfere with implanted electronic devices, and (c) electrocautery does not carry the risk of alternate site burn that may potentially be seen with electrosurgery at the site of the return electrode or when an electrode wire or surgical table comes in contact with patient's body. Therefore, electrocautery may be the preferred tool in the hands of inexperienced operators and may not need the extensive training needed for electrosurgery.

Hot wire electrocautery can be used for the destruction of epidermal lesions such as warts or for hemostasis of bleeding surfaces. For the destruction of deeper dermis or a deep destruction of any tissue, the superficial burned tissues can be removed using a tool such as a curette after the first pass of cautery. Then the procedure can be repeated. Keeping the hot wire in contact with tissue may cause a relatively deep burn and tissue destruction; however, the final depth of destruction is not easy to predict during the procedure.

Electrosurgical devices usually have higher power than electrocautery devices. Therefore, they are preferred to electrocautery when the surface area of the target is large. Electrosurgical devices are also preferred to electrocautery when the target area is very small. Needle-shaped electrosurgical electrodes can concentrate the current on a very small area, smaller than the contact area of most electrocautery devices.

2.3 History of Electrosurgery

The concept of using heat for hemostasis dates back hundreds, if not thousands, of years. As technology evolved, devices were developed that used electricity to heat tissue and control bleeding, laying the groundwork for modern-day electrosurgery.

Electricity was first used in surgery in the early nineteenth century when French physicist Becquerel used hot wire electrocautery. He passed a direct current through a metallic wire to make it hot. He then applied the hot wire to the tissue to thermally cauterize it.

In 1881, a French biophysicist named D'Arsonval discovered that high-frequency alternating currents could pass through the human and animal body and generate heat without causing painful electrical shock or muscle stimulation. This discovery helped scientists to conduct more studies in this field and develop modern electrosurgery.

Between 1890 and 1910, Nagelschmidt, a German physician, introduced the concept of diathermy. He used two large surface electrodes, larger than the return electrodes used in modern electrosurgery, to pass a high-frequency electrical current through an extremity, warming it in the process. He explained how high-frequency electrical currents and high-frequency electromagnetic fields can create heat in the body through the agitation and vibration of molecules. Modern microwave ovens in our houses use practically the same mechanism to heat our food.

Nagelschmidt used diathermy for therapeutic purposes and found that patients with articular and circulatory problems may benefit from the application of this method. A few years later, Czerny used the heating effect of high-frequency electrical currents for cutting tissue. He used a setting similar to the cutting mode of current electrosurgical devices. He also referred to his method as diathermy. Because of this, the word diathermy was originally used to encompass both medical diathermy (therapeutic heating technique) and surgical diathermy (electrosection). While some still use the term diathermy today to describe electrosurgery, the more accurate and preferred term is electrosurgery. It's also worth noting that medical diathermy for therapeutic heating is now largely obsolete in clinical practice.

In 1900, a French physician, Joseph Rivere, observed coagulation of tissue as a result of a spark arcing from a diathermy electrode. He subsequently used this arcing current to treat a carcinomatous ulcer on a patient's hand. This event has been cited as the first true therapeutic use of electrosurgery in medicine.

During the early 1900s, Simon Pozzi used high-frequency, high-voltage, low-amperage currents to treat skin cancers in a technique he termed fulguration. Doyen introduced a patient return electrode to increase the power of the device and the depth of destruction. He named his method electrocoagulation and used it primarily for hemostasis.

Around 1910, William Clark started using a high-amperage, low-voltage current to produce shorter sparks. He observed under a microscope that tissues subjected to this current shrunk from dehydration. He used the term desiccation to describe the effect when tissues were destroyed by this dehydration.

In the late 1920s, a collaboration between physicist William T. Bovie and neurosurgeon Harvey Cushing resulted in the development of the predecessor of today's electrosurgical units. The new machine was able to offer coagulation during cutting, with effective hemostasis on the incision walls. It helped the surgeon reduce bleeding during surgery for vascular brain tumors and resulted in better outcomes. Bovie's electrosurgical generator was the first commercially available electrosurgical device on the market. This electrosurgical unit model was used until 1968, when other models were developed by other manufacturers.

Previous generations of electrosurgical generators used a spark gap and/or a vacuum tube to make high-frequency electrosurgical currents. To generate a high-voltage, low-amperage current for electrofulguration, these devices used damped currents characterized by a high ratio of peak-to-average voltage. Modern electrosurgical units use transistors to make high-frequency currents with a variety of waveforms. Interrupted waves produced by modern devices have replaced damped currents and have the same effect and properties as damped currents in older devices.

2.4 Skin Structure and Wound Healing

2.4.1 Skin Anatomy

Skin is composed of three layers: epidermis, dermis, and subcutaneous fat. The outermost layer, the epidermis, forms the main barrier between the body and the environment. The second layer, the dermis, provides the most physical support to the skin.

2.4.1.1 Epidermis

The outermost layer of the skin is called the epidermis. Epidermis is a self-regenerating layer of stratified squamous epithelium varying in thickness from 0.04 mm on the eyelids and genitalia to 1.5 mm on the palms and soles.

The stratum corneum is the outermost layer of the epidermis. This layer consists of dead cells (corneocytes) that form a very effective barrier to protect underlying tissue from infection, dehydration, chemicals, and mechanical stress. The stratum corneum is very thick on the palms and soles, and where there is a callosity. When this layer is dry, it shows relatively high electrical resistance, especially to direct currents.

The deepest keratinocytes on dermoepidermal junction are called basal cells. Basal keratinocytes are active proliferative stem cells that continuously proliferate and make new keratinocytes. These cells are in charge of building new cells for epidermal repair after any damage to the epidermis such as wounds or burns.

2.4.1.2 Dermis

The dermis is a flexible network of collagen and elastin fibers embedded in a ground substance matrix that accommodates fibroblasts, immune systems, neuronal cells, lymphatic channels, and vasculature.

The dermis varies in thickness from 0.5 mm on the eyelid to more than 4.0 mm on the back. This layer can be divided into two layers. The thin upper layer is called the papillary layer. This layer is composed of thin, haphazardly arranged collagen fibers. The thicker lower layer is called the reticular layer and extends from the base of the papillary layer to the subcutaneous tissue. This deeper layer is composed of thick collagen fibers.

2.4.1.3 Epidermal Appendages: Adnexa

Eccrine, apocrine, and sebaceous glands, as well as hair follicles, originate as downgrowth from the epidermis into the dermis. While these various adnexal structures serve specific functions, they all can function as reserve epidermal cells for repair of superficial epidermis after injury. If a superficial partial-thickness wound such as a second-degree burn destructs the epidermis, but not deeper dermis, basal cells in epidermal appendages in the dermis start replicating and migrate toward the surface to participate in the reepithelialization of the surface and wound healing. Skin sites such as the face or scalp which contain more pilosebaceous units reepithelialize more rapidly than skin sites such as the back, where adnexae of all types are comparatively scarce.

2.4.2 Wound Healing and Scar Formation

Wounds can be divided based on the depth of injury. Full-thickness wounds involve the whole epidermis and dermis, down to subcutaneous fat. Superficial partial-thickness wounds happen after the loss of epidermis and maybe papillary dermis. A deep partial-thickness wound is the loss of epidermis, papillary dermis, and some reticular dermis.

If a wound is left open to heal by secondary intension, the epidermal cells need to replicate and migrate to cover the wound's surface. Full-thickness wounds heal from periphery by the epidermal cells migrating from the surrounding skin. However, in partial-thickness wounds, the adnexa in the deeper dermis in the wound bed provide epidermal cells to migrate and cover the wound at the same time the surrounding skin is providing migratory epidermal cells.

While loss of epidermis and papillary dermis may heal without scar formation, scaring happens when there is significant damage to or change in the structure of reticular dermis. Therefore, all full-thickness and most deep partial-thickness wounds result in scar formation.

Superficial partial-thickness wounds may not result in scars if we can protect reticular dermis against further damage from drying, infection, or inflammation. An appropriate dressing providing a moist wound environment can protect reticular dermis while providing a good environment for epidermal cells to replicate and migrate and cover the dermis. Excessive inflammation in the wound can result in changes in the dermal architecture and scar formation. The sooner a superficial partial-thickness wound epithelializes and heals, the less is the chance of scar formation from inflammatory damage in reticular dermis.

Even after epithelialization of the wound, an abnormal inflammatory process may continue in the skin and may result in the formation of hypertrophic scars. Any significant inflammation (deep red color) in the skin after reepithelialization necessitates urgent treatment to prevent dermal changes from abnormal inflammation. Using superpotent topical glucocorticoids plus tretinoin can prevent scar formation in this setting [1]. Intralesional injection of long-acting glucocorticoids is another option for smaller areas.

Reference

1. Taheri A, Moradi Tuchayi S, Alinia H, Orscheln CS, Mansoori P, Feldman SR. Topical clobetasol in conjunction with topical tretinoin is effective in preventing scar formation after superficial partial-thickness burn ulcers of the skin: a retrospective study. J Dermatol Treat. 2015;26(4):361–4. https://doi.org/10.3109/09546634.2014.991677. PubMed PMID: 25424054.

Chapter 3
Fundamentals of Electricity as Applied to Electrosurgery

Abstract

- When an electrical current (direct or alternating) passes through an organism's body, tissue resistance to the flow of electricity converts electrical energy to heat.
- A direct or low-frequency current can cause a chemical reaction called electrolysis at the electrode–tissue interface where the current enters or exits the body. The chemical effects of electrolysis diminish at higher frequencies.
- A direct or low-frequency alternating current can depolarize cell membranes and cause neuromuscular excitation. Neuromuscular stimulation becomes negligible at higher frequencies.
- In a high-frequency alternating current circuit, cables and pathways of electricity inherently form capacitors with each other and with nearby conductive environmental objects. Therefore, all insulation on instruments and cables is relative, and some energy always leaks through it as a capacitive current.

3.1 Electricity and Electrical Currents

An electric current is produced when a power supply provides energy to a circuit, which is a closed path that allows electricity to flow. The power supply creates a potential difference (voltage). This potential difference exerts a force on the free charge carriers (electrons or ions) in the circuit and pushes them around toward the opposite terminal of the power source. The rate of flow of these charge-carrying particles is called electric current, and it is measured in amperes (amps).

Opposition to the flow of the current in the circuit is called resistance or impedance, measured in ohms. The resistance of an object is proportional to the length of the object and its resistivity and inversely proportional to its cross-sectional area. A material's resistivity refers to its inherent capacity to resist electric current. A copper wire has a lower resistivity than a cotton rope. A shorter copper wire has less resistance than a longer one. A metallic wire with a larger diameter has less resistance than a thinner one with the same length.

A. Taheri et al., *Advanced Electrosurgery*,
https://doi.org/10.1007/978-3-032-28342-9_3

The human body contains different tissues which all have varying resistivity. Tissues with lower water content, such as fat and bone, have high resistivity, while muscle and blood, which contain more water, have low resistivity. In the skin, the epidermis resists current more than the dermis, but a moist, well-hydrated epidermis has lower resistivity than dry epidermis.

When electric current flows through a resistance, heat is produced. The power generated, measured in watts (W), represents the energy produced per second. The flow of a current follows Ohm's law:

$$V = I \times R,$$

where V = voltage, I = amperage, and R = resistance.

Power can also be expressed as $P = V^2/R$. Thus, a high-voltage source with low resistance produces a high current and high power. However, every electrical generator or battery has a maximum power output. If the circuit's resistance becomes too low, the generator may be unable to sustain its output, causing the overall power delivered to decrease (Fig. 3.1).

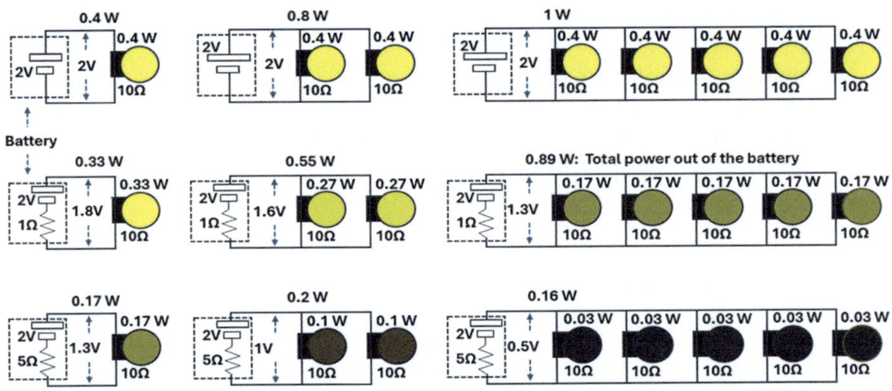

Fig. 3.1 A simple circuit consisting of a 2-volt battery connected to 10-ohm light bulbs. The nominal voltage of a battery is its open-circuit voltage, which is the voltage when there is nothing connected to it and there is no current flowing. Once a load is added, the terminal voltage drops because some energy is lost across the battery's internal resistance. The higher this internal resistance, the greater the voltage drops and the lower the power available to load. Batteries or generators with low internal resistance can deliver higher power with minimal voltage loss. Top: An *ideal* battery with no internal resistance. An ideal 2-volt battery delivers a steady 2 V regardless of the load. One 10-ohm bulb receives 0.4 W of power ($0.4 = 2^2/10$). Adding more bulbs does not reduce the voltage, so each bulb stays equally bright, and the total power output increases. Middle: With a 1Ω internal resistance, the 2-volt battery's terminal voltage drops slightly as more bulbs are added. Since higher current flows through the internal resistance, part of the voltage is lost inside the battery. Although the total power drawn from the battery increases with more bulbs, each bulb gets less voltage and therefore appears dimmer than with an ideal battery. Bottom: A small 2-volt battery with 5Ω internal resistance loses more energy inside the battery itself. Even powering a single bulb is difficult, and connecting several bulbs causes a large voltage drop. As a result, the bulbs receive very little current and produce very dim light or none at all

There are two main types of electrical current: direct current and alternating current. Direct current (DC) flows in one constant direction through a simple circuit. Batteries are common sources of DC power.

Alternating current (AC), on the other hand, reverses direction periodically. Household wall outlets, for example, supply AC power. In AC, both voltage and current fluctuate between zero and a maximum value (peak voltage) during each cycle (Fig. 3.2).

For AC circuits, the effective voltage, also called the root mean square (RMS) voltage, is used to describe the power delivered. RMS voltage is lower than the peak voltage and represents the equivalent DC voltage that would produce the same heating or power effect. For example, a lamp connected to a 6-V RMS AC supply will shine just as brightly as it would on a steady 6-V DC supply (Fig. 3.2).

In the United States, household wall outlets provide 110-V AC. This 110 V refers to the RMS voltage, meaning the actual voltage fluctuates between zero and values higher than 110 V (Fig. 3.2).

For direct current, electricity flows only when there is a continuous conductive path. If the circuit is broken, current cannot flow. In contrast, alternating current can sometimes pass across small gaps or insulation through mechanisms such as capacitance.

A capacitor is formed when two conductive plates are placed close together but separated by a nonconductive material (Fig. 3.3). When AC voltage is applied, the changing electric field causes a current to effectively "pass" through the capacitor, even though there is no direct conductive connection. This is called a capacitive current. Importantly, higher-frequency AC currents pass through capacitors more easily than lower-frequency signals, making frequency an important factor in how AC behaves in capacitive circuits.

In an alternating current circuit, cables and conductive pathways naturally form capacitors with each other and with nearby conductive objects. Because of this, high-frequency AC cannot be perfectly insulated. Even with protective coatings, some energy always leaks through as capacitive current. In electrosurgery, this leakage can lead to energy loss or even patient burns if not properly managed.

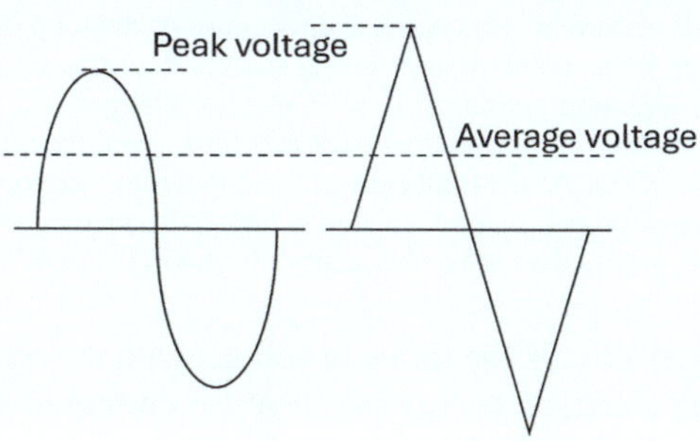

Fig. 3.2 Peak and average voltage of alternating electrical currents. In AC waveforms, the peak voltage is the maximum value reached during each cycle, while the average (effective) voltage is lower. The ratio of peak voltage to average voltage is called the crest factor. A lower crest factor means the waveform has smaller peaks relative to its average voltage. In electrosurgery, generators with lower crest factors produce smaller sparks and cleaner cuts

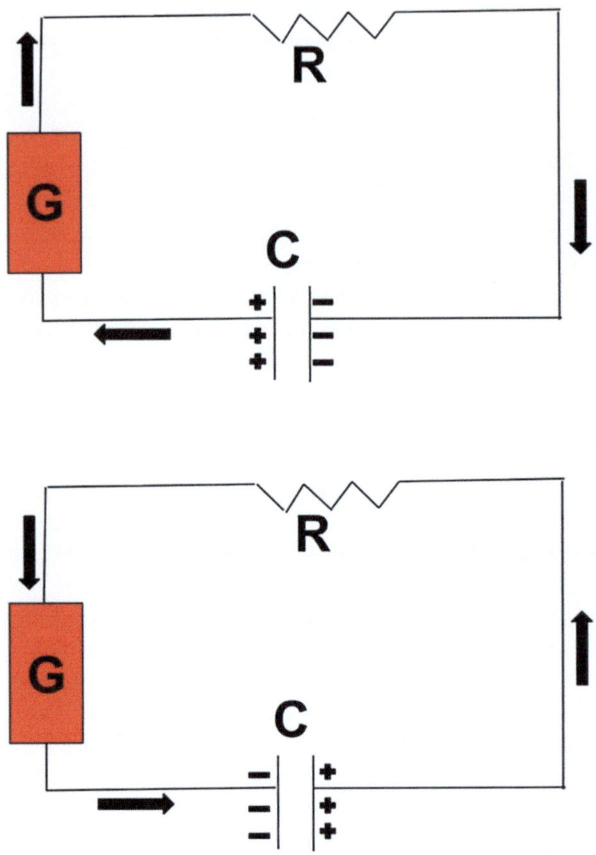

Fig. 3.3 An alternate current circuit with a generator (G), a resistor (R), and a capacitor (C). A capacitor consists of two conductive plates separated by a nonconductive material. When a direct current voltage source is applied, there is an initial surge of current as electrons accumulate on one plate, giving it a negative charge, while electrons leave the other plate, making it positively charged. During this brief charging period, current flows for only a fraction of a second. Once the capacitor is fully charged, the flow of current stops because direct current cannot pass through the insulating layer anymore. However, with an alternating current source, the situation is different. Since alternating current reverses direction periodically, the capacitor charges and discharges during each cycle. This allows a capacitive current to flow back and forth, even though there is no direct conductive path between the plates. As the frequency of the alternating current increases, more current passes through the capacitor per second, meaning higher-frequency alternating current flows through a capacitor more easily than lower-frequency alternating current

In an electrosurgery circuit, the tissue in contact with the active electrode acts as a resistor, converting electrical energy into heat for cutting or coagulation. Ideally, current should only enter the body at the point where the active electrode touches the tissue. However, if the active electrode cable comes into contact with the patient's skin, a capacitor may form between the cable and the patient's body. This allows some current to pass through the cable's insulation and enter the patient at an unintended site (Fig. 3.4). If a high-power generator remains active for a prolonged period, this leakage current can cause unwanted patient burns [1].

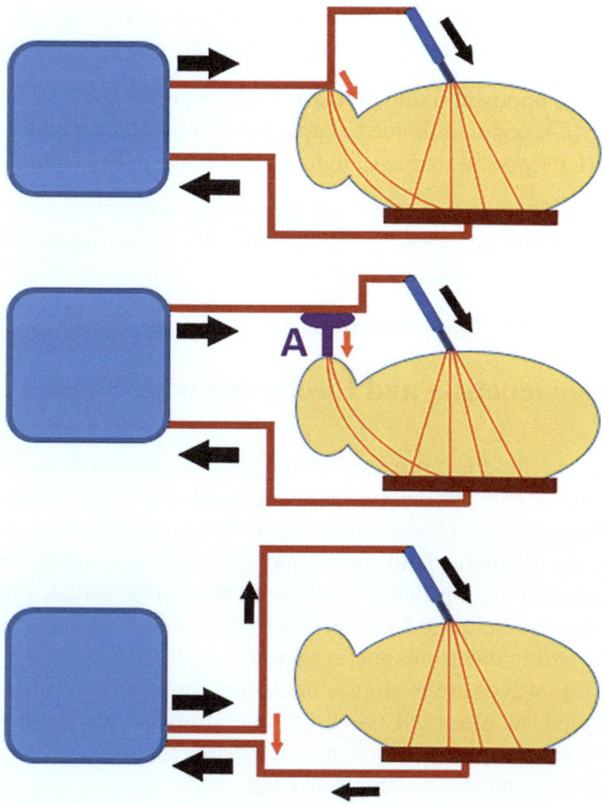

Fig. 3.4 Current leakage in electrosurgery circuit. If the active electrode cable is placed too close to the patient's body, some capacitive current may pass through the cable's insulation and enter the patient at an unintended site, potentially causing a burn (top). Leakage can also occur if the active cable is near a conductive object that is in contact or close to the patient or surgical staff (middle). Examples include a surgical table or a metal clamp used to secure the cable to surgical drapes. The current can flow through these objects, creating a risk of unintended burns. If the active and return electrode cables are placed near each other, current can leak from the active cable to the return cable before reaching the patient (bottom). This reduces the current delivered to the tissue, meaning the power dissipated in the patient is lower than the generator's output

Current leakage can also occur between the active electrode cable and the return electrode cable. If the two cables are placed too close together, or near a conductive object, a capacitor forms between them. Some current then bypasses the patient's body, flowing directly from the active cable to the return cable (Fig. 3.4). This reduces the available current at the active electrode and at the surgical site, potentially affecting performance and efficiency.

As mentioned earlier, higher-frequency alternating currents pass through capacitors more easily than lower-frequency currents and are harder to insulate. Ultrahigh frequencies above 5 MHz are rarely used in electrosurgery because leakage currents may exceed safety limits [2].

While resistance opposes the flow of direct current in a circuit, the opposition to alternating current (AC) is called impedance. Impedance is composed of:

- Resistance (R): opposition due to resistive elements
- Capacitance (C): opposition due to capacitors, known as capacitive reactance
- Inductance (L): opposition due to inductors or coils, called inductive reactance

Unlike resistors, capacitors and inductors do not convert electrical energy into heat; they only oppose AC flow. In electrosurgical circuits, inductive reactance is negligible and will not be discussed further.

3.2 Electromagnetism and Electromagnetic Fields

An electromagnetic field is a property of space associated with the motion of electric charges (electric currents). A stationary charged particle produces only an electric field, while a moving charge generates both an electric field and a magnetic field. A changing magnetic field can induce an electric current, and similarly a changing electric field can produce a magnetic field. The mutual interaction of an electric and magnetic field produces an electromagnetic field that can be described as a wave transporting electromagnetic energy.

Light and radio waves are examples of electromagnetic waves. Electromagnetic fields exist around all electrical wires and are stronger near high-voltage power lines. Devices such as microwave ovens use intense electromagnetic waves to heat food by transferring energy to water molecules.

3.3 Electrical Conduction in Biological Tissues

Electrical conduction depends on the type of conductive material. In metals, the charge carriers are primarily electrons. In gases and liquids, the carriers are ions. Gases are usually nonconductive. However, when exposed to a high-voltage electric field (e.g., between the poles of a high-voltage generator), the gas becomes ionized, forming a plasma that conducts current as a spark. Examples include lightning in nature and fulguration in electrosurgery.

Alternating electromagnetic fields can transfer energy through materials that are normally nonconductive under DC. One common mechanism is polarization of atoms or molecules. For example, in a microwave oven, water molecules in food are polarized and absorb energy, causing the food to heat. In polarization, charges do not leave their molecules as they do in a conductor. Instead, electrons shift slightly toward the positive pole of the field, and protons toward the negative pole. Each time the electromagnetic field changes direction, the molecules reorient, conducting a small, temporary amount of energy. With alternating fields, this process occurs repeatedly. The higher the frequency, the more energy passes per unit time. Microwave ovens use gigahertz-range alternating electromagnetic fields, producing enough energy to warm food efficiently. There are different forms of polarization. Figures 3.5 and 3.6 show the most common forms of polarization.

When an electrical current passes through biological tissue, polarization can occur. With direct current, conduction is mainly ionic, occurring through extracellular fluids, because cell membranes act as insulators and block DC flow. High-frequency currents, such as those used in electrosurgery, can cross cell membranes via capacitive currents and polarization. Once inside a cell, current can continue flowing through the ionic interior and exit through the membrane again via the same mechanisms. Overall, electrical conduction through tissue occurs through multiple parallel pathways, combining ionic conductors with serial and parallel capacitive elements formed by cell membranes. This complex structure allows high-frequency currents to penetrate tissues more effectively than direct currents. Tissues with a high cell density and low extracellular fluid, such as the epidermis, behave like multiple capacitors with few conductive pathways. These tissues resist direct current but allow high-frequency alternating currents to pass more easily through capacitive or polarization mechanisms.

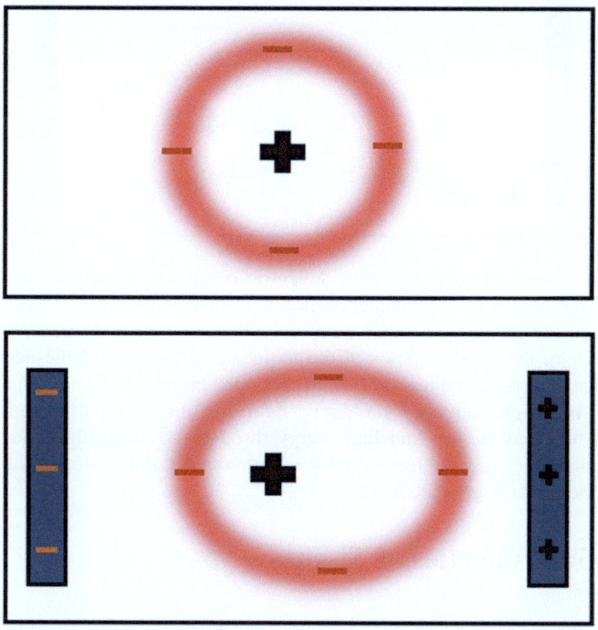

Fig. 3.5 *Dielectric polarization* occurs when a dielectric material is placed in an electromagnetic field. Each atom in the material consists of a positively charged nucleus surrounded by a cloud of electrons (top). When an electric field is applied, the electron cloud is slightly pulled toward the positive pole of the field, distorting the atom (bottom). This creates a separation of charge, with one side more negative and the opposite side more positive, forming an atomic dipole. In a direct current or constant field, the atoms remain polarized without motion, so there is no significant flow of current or energy. In an alternating electromagnetic field, the field repeatedly changes direction. The dipoles reorient rapidly with each change, allowing a small current or energy transfer each time the polarity reverses

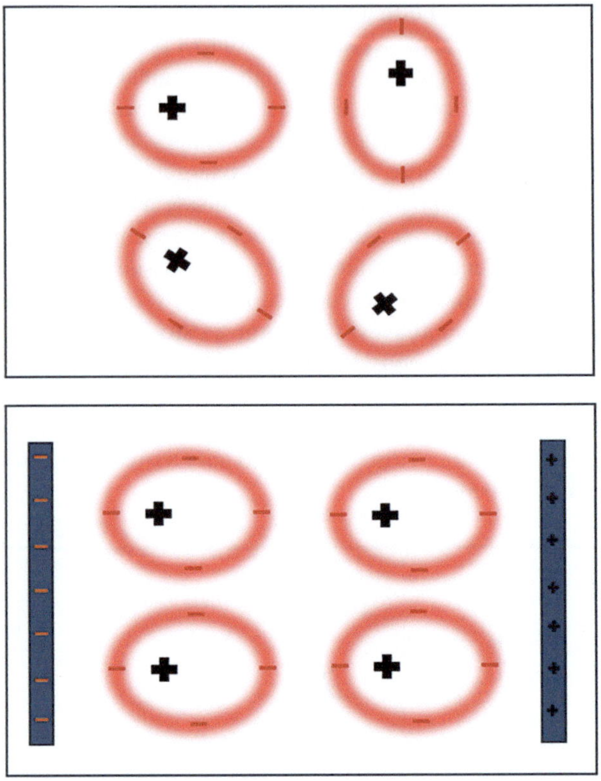

Fig. 3.6 *Dipolar polarization* is similar to dielectric polarization, but in this case the material already contains molecules with permanent dipoles. In their natural state, these dipoles are randomly oriented, so the material is unpolarized overall (top). When the material is placed in an electromagnetic field, the positive poles of the molecules align toward the negative pole of the field, and the negative poles align toward the positive pole, polarizing the material as a whole (bottom). If the field is a high-frequency alternating field, the dipoles rapidly change direction with each cycle. This repeated motion transfers energy through the material, producing heating. For example, water molecules in a microwave oven vibrate rapidly in the alternating electromagnetic field, generating heat that warms the food

3.4 Electric Properties of Tissues

The electrical properties of biological tissues determine the pathways of current flow through the body and the effect of the currents on tissues.

The electrical properties of each organ can depend on the tissue types present in the organ, tissue temperature, hydration, type of extracellular materials, tissue orientation relative to the applied current or electromagnetic field, and the frequency of the applied current or field.

At low frequencies, the biological tissues will behave practically like a conductor. However, capacitive and polarization effects will become more important at higher frequencies. Skin is a highly heterogeneous structure, which thus leads to heterogeneous resistivity and polarization. The epidermis is the outer layer of skin. The thickness of the epidermis varies in different types of skin. It is the thinnest on the eyelids and the thickest on the palms and soles. The epidermis is made of epidermal cells tightly attached with minimal extracellular fluid between the cells. The lack of significant extracellular fluid in the epidermis makes this layer relatively resistant to the flow of direct currents. High-frequency alternating currents can flow through this layer more easily than direct currents using capacitive effect and polarization. The stratum corneum is the outermost layer of the epidermis, consisting of dead and usually dehydrated cells. Although this dry dead layer is very thin, it has a high resistivity to direct current and high impedance to alternating currents. A hydrated or wet epidermis has lower resistance and impedance to electrical currents.

At a low-frequency range (under 10 kHz), the impedance of the skin is dominated by the stratum corneum even though this layer is very thin. At frequencies around 10 kHz, the share of stratum corneum in the total impedance of skin may be around 50% depending on the thickness of the stratum corneum, and at 100 kHz, this share may drop to around 10% if the epidermis is thin [3]. A reduction in impedance is observed in practically all biological tissues between the frequency of 10 kHz and 100 kHz; however, this reduction is more significant in tissues that have less extracellular fluid and more cell membranes and therefore are more dependent on capacitive effect and polarization for passing alternative currents.

Bone and fat have the highest resistivity among the internal organs, while blood vessels, nerves, and muscles have relatively lower resistance. The skeletal muscles have lower resistance when the current passes longitudinally along the muscle fibers, compared with when the current passes transversely or vertically to the fibers. The reason is that skeletal muscle cells are long, tube-shaped cells. Therefore, when the current passes along the fibers, it can use the ionic conductivity of the intracellular fluid inside the long tubes and does not have to pass through multiple cell walls [4].

3.5 Chemical Effects of Electrical Currents on Tissues

When a direct current enters an electrolyte or our body through a metallic electrode, a chemical reaction called *electrolysis* occurs at the electrode–tissue interface.

In electrolysis, each electrode attracts ions that are of the opposite charge. Positively charged ions (cations) move toward the electron-providing negative electrode and receive electrons. Negatively charged ions (anions) move toward the electron-extracting positive electrode and give up their electrons. On the other hand, when neutral atoms or molecules that are in contact with the surface of an electrode gain or lose electrons, they become ions and may dissolve in the electrolyte and react with other ions or substances. These chemical reactions at the electrode–tissue interface may destroy a thin layer of tissue around the electrode.

Electrolysis has been used as a method of hair removal (galvanic depilation) and for the treatment of telangiectasia. In this method, a thin needle is introduced into the skin. Then, a low-power direct current is passed through the needle for a few seconds to minutes. The chemically damaged tissue around the needle may not show any color or consistency change at the time of the procedure; however, it undergoes necrosis in a few hours to days.

A low-frequency alternating current can also cause a chemical reaction similar to a direct current and can cause tissue damage. However, since the chemical reaction of each phase can be neutralized by the opposite phase, these chemical effects diminish as the frequency of alternations increases. Electrolysis effect and its chemical tissue damage almost disappear at frequencies higher than 5–10 kHz [5–11].

3.6 Effects of Electrical Currents on Cell Membranes

Neuronal and muscular cells in higher organisms maintain an internal environment that is negatively charged relative to the cell's exterior. This difference in charge is called *cell membrane resting potential*. Some signals to these cells from other neurons open some channels in the cell membrane that let the positively charged ions such as sodium or calcium rush into the cell and change the negative internal charge of the cell temporarily to positive. This shift from a negative to a positive membrane potential is called depolarization or an action potential. During an action potential or depolarization, the nerves can send a signal to the surrounding neurons or muscles and stimulate them as well. Nerve stimulation may cause a range of feelings such as pain or tingling. Depolarization of muscles causes muscle contraction.

Low-voltage currents lower than 24 V that are used in cars and trucks are generally safe and cannot cause significant neuromuscular excitation if they are applied to our skin. Currents with voltages higher than 40 V can cause neuromuscular excitation, especially if the skin is moist.

Direct currents and low-frequency alternate currents cannot pass through the tissue if just one pole of the battery or generator comes in contact with the skin. The current needs to have a path to go back to the generator, or it is not a current. If we touch the active (live) wires that carry electricity in our household with one finger, we probably do not feel anything. However, if we touch the other wire with the other hand at the same time, or if our foot is on a wet or electrically conductive floor, the current has a path to flow through our body to the other wire or the earth. And this flowing current can cause neuromuscular excitation along its path.

A direct current applied to the tissue can depolarize cell membranes and cause neuromuscular excitation. When this direct current is sustained for a period of time, the cells enter a refractory period wherein neuromuscular excitation ceases. On the other hand, low-frequency alternate currents such as electric power in our houses can cause severe neuromuscular excitation and tetanic muscular contraction because they do not induce a refractory period. In other words, low-frequency alternate currents can cause more severe neuromuscular excitation than direct currents.

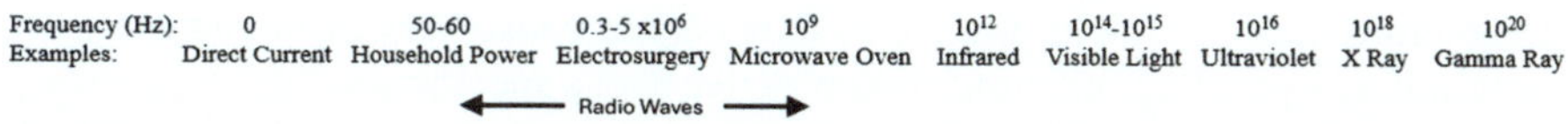

Fig. 3.7 Electromagnetic spectrum. Electrosurgical units use alternating currents with frequencies that are part of the radio-wave frequency range

Neuromuscular stimulation associated with alternating currents decreases as the frequency of current increases above 1 kHz and becomes negligible at frequencies of 100–300 kHz [6, 7, 11, 12]. At these high frequencies, current reversal is so rapid that cellular ion position change is essentially nil, and depolarization fails to occur. High-frequency alternating currents thus make it possible to exploit the heating effects of electricity while avoiding the undesirable neuromuscular effects. Whereas physiological reasons dictate the lower limit of the frequency employed, as detailed earlier, practical and safety considerations regarding current leakage place restrictions on the upper limit of the current frequency used in electrosurgical units. Electrosurgical units usually produce alternating currents with a frequency of 0.3–5 MHz. These frequencies are part of the radio-wave frequency range (Fig. 3.7), hence the reason electrosurgery is also called "radiofrequency (RF) surgery" or "high-frequency electrosurgery."

3.7 Thermal Effects of Electrical Currents on Tissues

Low-voltage or low-power electrical currents may cause electrolysis and/or neuromuscular excitation; however, they may not be able to produce significant heat in tissues to cause thermal damage. Higher voltages such as 110–240 V of household power or higher can pass easier through the tissue and cause significant burns. The main barrier to the entrance or exit of electricity to or from the body is usually the epidermis on the skin which has the highest resistance to the passage of electricity. A wet or hydrated epidermis has less resistance to electricity, passes the electrical currents better, and can cause more severe electrical shock. A high-voltage current can cause skin burns at the site of current entrance into the body and also at the site of exit from the body. A very-high-voltage or very-high-power current may cause a more extensive burn all along its path in the body. Because muscles and vessels have less resistance against the passage of electrical currents, currents preferentially flow through these tissues and burn them preferentially. Victims of electrical burns that have two or more burned spots on their skin (likely one entrance and one exit) may have deeper vascular or muscle injuries and need to be evaluated and may be observed in a hospital. Damaged muscle cells may release a protein called myoglobin into the blood (rhabdomyolysis) that can precipitate in the kidneys and cause kidney failure, if not treated.

Electrosurgical devices provide enough power output for achieving thermal changes in a small volume of tissue in the vicinity of the active electrode. Their maximum output is limited; therefore, they cannot cause very deep and extensive burns, unless a very large electrode is kept active over a specific area for a long period.

With a current passing through tissue, an increase in temperature below the boiling point can cause irreversible damage to the tissue materials, especially proteins. This change results in cell death and a change in tissue consistency. This process is called *coagulation*. The higher the temperature, the sooner coagulation happens. In the skin, different tissues react differently to this thermal injury and have different consistencies after coagulation. Consistency change in these tissues mainly depends on their collagen (one of the skin proteins) concentration. The epidermis and superficial (papillary) dermis do not have a high concentration of collagen. These tissues turn to a soft doughy material (liquefaction) that can be wiped off the skin using gauze or a blunt curette after coagulation. In contrast, the deep (reticular) dermis, which has a high concentration of collagen, turns into a firm tissue and contracts immediately after coagulation [13]. This firm coagulated material cannot be wiped off easily. In order to remove this firm layer, a sharp curette is needed. This difference in the consistency of the tissues upon coagulation helps the surgeons to differentiate the papillary dermis from the reticular dermis and avoid deep tissue damage and potential scars when the target lesion is just in the epidermis or superficial dermis.

Adipose tissue including subcutaneous fat has a low concentration of proteins, and therefore it reacts to an increase in temperature differently. Adipocytes or fat cells in subcutaneous tissue usually burst upon coagulation. And since there is not much extracellular matrix as structural support between adipocytes, electrosurgery may cut through the adipose tissue even when the goal is to coagulate.

3.8 Entrance and Propagation Pattern of High-Frequency Electrical Currents in Biological Tissues

When an electrical current passes through a wire or a cylindrical conductor such as a finger, the current density will be the same through its path in the wire or cylinder. However, when a relatively small electrode applies an electrical current to a small point on the surface of a large piece of homogenous tissue, the current spreads and propagates in all directions in the tissue mass (Fig. 3.8). Current spread causes the current density to fall and have less thermal effect with distance from the electrode.

Although there is a clear correlation between the frequency of current and the pattern of its movement in long wire-shaped conductors (skin effect), in vitro studies on electrosurgical currents could not find any relation between the frequency of current and its propagation pattern in biological tissues [14].

The entrance and propagation pattern of electrosurgical currents in tissues depends not only on the tissue itself but also on the shape of the electrode and the electrode–tissue interface. When a large-tip active electrode is used, the current prefers to concentrate on the periphery or the extremities of the electrode and to enter

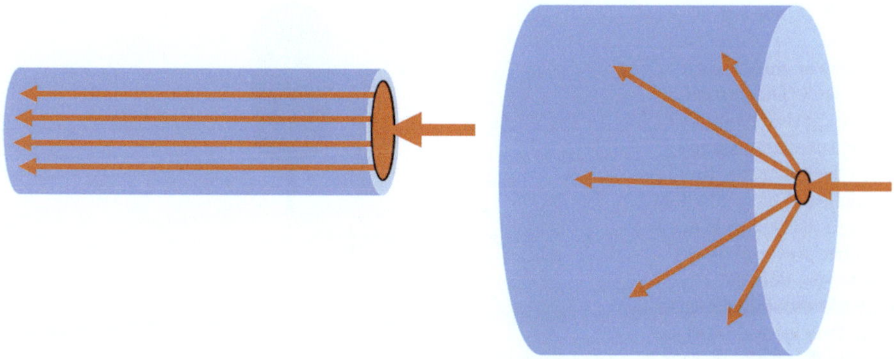

Fig. 3.8 When an electrical current passes through a cylindrical conductor, the current density will be the same through its path. However, when a small electrode applies an electrical current to the surface of a large mass, the current spreads, leading to a fall in current density with distance from the electrode

preferentially into the tissue in contact with those areas. Therefore, current density and heating effect may not be the same in all tissues in contact with the active electrode or in all directions around the electrode.

3.8.1 Propagation Pattern of Electrical Currents When Using a Fine-Tip Active Electrode

A fine-tip active electrode can have a small electrode–tissue interface and can concentrate a current on a fine point in tissue adjacent to its tip. When using a fine-tip electrode, the current density in tissue rapidly decreases with distance from the electrode (Fig. 3.9); therefore, heat generation is practically confined to the vicinity of the electrode tip, potentially limiting the depth of thermal tissue effect [15].

3.8.2 Propagation Pattern of Electrical Currents When Using a Large-Tip Active Electrode

When an electrode with a large electrode–tissue interface is used, the current may prefer to use specific paths and preferentially enter the tissue from specific points on the contact area. This may cause nonhomogeneous coagulation at the electrode–tissue interface. The reason is that charged particles of the same polarity (positive versus negative) in any object tend to be as far apart as possible, rather than being homogeneously distributed. Therefore, the net electric charge of a conductor resides entirely on its surface, with more charges on the extremities of the object [16].

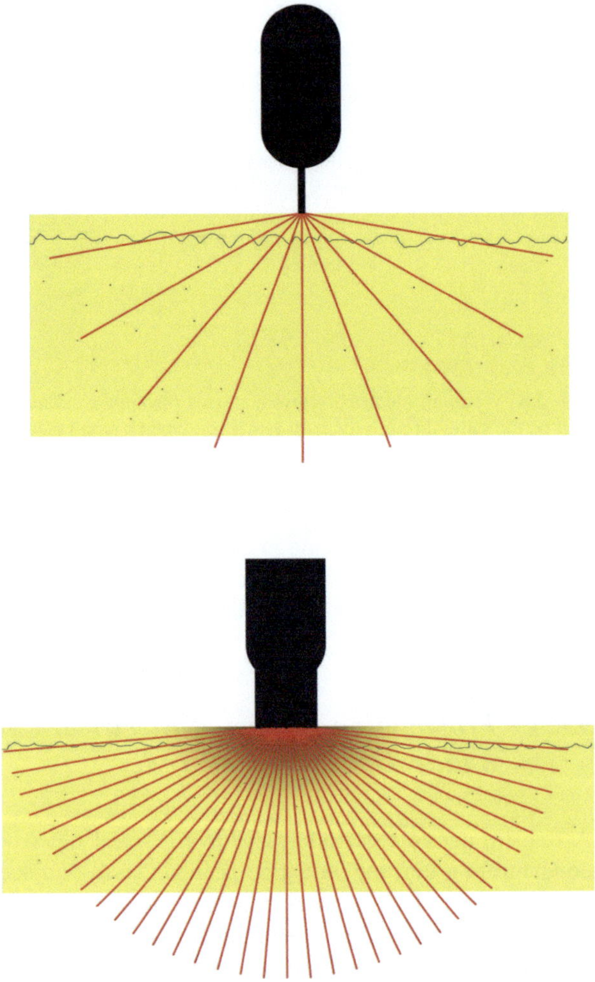

Fig. 3.9 A fine-tip electrode can concentrate a low-power current on a small area. The current density in tissue rapidly decreases with distance from the electrode, limiting the depth of thermal effect. A large-tip electrode needs a higher power to work; the current density decreases with distance from the electrode surface slowly; therefore, there is a higher current concentration in deeper layers of tissue compared with when using a fine-tip electrode

In a cylindrical electrosurgical electrode or an electrode with a disk-shaped head, most of the charge will be concentrated on the perimeter of the electrode. If the disk-shaped end of this electrode comes in contact with tissue (a disk-shaped electrode–tissue interface), the periphery of the electrode–tissue contact area will receive the highest current density. Therefore, thermal damage in tissue starts from the periphery of the contact area along the perimeter of the electrode (Fig. 3.10) [17]. With continuing the application of the current, gradually all the contact area is coagulated (Fig. 3.10). Interestingly, the coagulation that starts on the periphery of the electrode–tissue contact area spreads deep in an arc-shaped pattern in a way that the tissue in contact with the center of the electrode experiences coagulation later than deeper tissue (Fig. 3.10) [17]. One explanation for this observation may be the cooling effect of the electrode. One should remember that, during electrocoagulation, heat generation occurs within the tissue while the active electrode acts as a conductor and remains cooler than the treated tissue [9]. And because the metallic electrode is a good heat conductor, it may prevent temperature rise in tissue near the

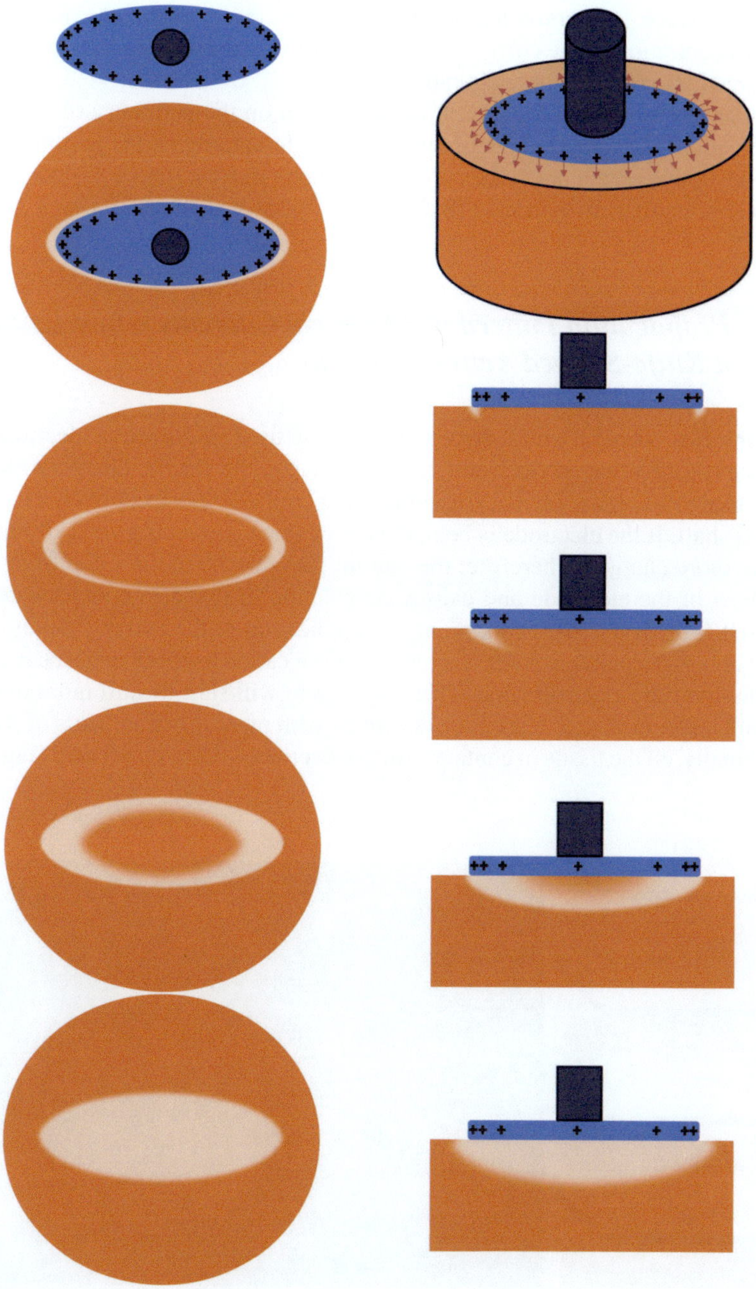

Fig. 3.10 Contact coagulation using an active electrode with a disk-shaped head. When a cylindrical or disk-shaped active electrosurgical electrode is used, most of the charge will be concentrated on the perimeter of the electrode. Therefore, the perimeter of the electrode–tissue contact area will receive the highest current density and coagulate first. When using an elliptical electrode (left), the extremities of the ellipse around the vertices will receive more current density. By continuing the application of the current, the coagulated area spreads deep in an arc-shaped pattern, and finally all the contact area is coagulated [17]

electrode surface. The combination of this cooling effect of the electrode and the lower concentration of the current in the center of the contact area may be the cause of the arc-shaped pattern of coagulation.

Similar to electrosurgery, current concentration on the periphery of an external cardiac defibrillator electrode may cause burn preferentially on the periphery of the electrode–body contact area when applying a direct current (shock) to the chest for treatment of cardiac arrhythmia [18].

3.8.3 Propagation Pattern of Electrical Currents When Using a Knife-Shaped Active Electrode

When the flat side of a knife-shaped electrode is used as an active electrosurgical electrode (a knife-shaped electrode–tissue interface), the electric charge of the electrode concentrates more on its extremities and peripheries, especially on its tip, than along its shaft. If the electrode is bent, the elbow (bent part) acts as an extremity and receives more charges. Therefore, the current flows to the tissue more from the tip and elbow of the electrode and causes coagulation in tissue in contact with those areas first (Fig. 3.11). With continuing the application of the current, finally, all the contact area is coagulated. After coagulation, desiccation happens in tissue in contact with the tip of the electrode first. Then the current will shift toward more moist tissues with lower electrical resistance in contact with more proximal parts of the electrode. Finally, all the tissue in contact with the electrode will be desiccated (Fig. 3.11).

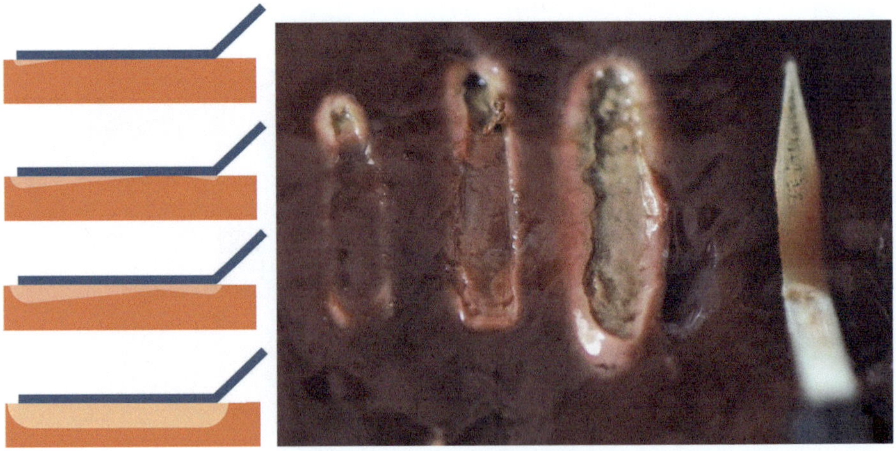

Fig. 3.11 Contact coagulation using the flat side of a knife-shaped electrode (a knife-shaped electrode–tissue interface). The electric charge of the electrode concentrates more on its extremities especially its tip and elbow (bent part) than along its shaft. With continuing the application of the current, coagulation starts in tissue in contact with those areas first, and then finally all the contact area is coagulated before desiccation happens

3.8.4 Propagation Pattern of Electrical Currents When Using a Penetrating Needle-Shaped Electrode

When a penetrating needle-shaped active electrode enters a large relatively homogenous mass of biological tissue, the maximum heating effect will be around the tip of the electrode in the deeper parts of the tissue (Fig. 3.12). As we discussed, the reason is that the electric charge of the needle resides more on its tip than along its shaft. With continuing the application of the current, finally, all the contact area is coagulated (Fig. 3.12) [19]. Penetrating needle-shaped electrodes have been used for electrocoagulation of deep targets while avoiding superficial tissues. Some devices use proximally insulated needle-shaped electrodes to direct the current to deeper tissue even better.

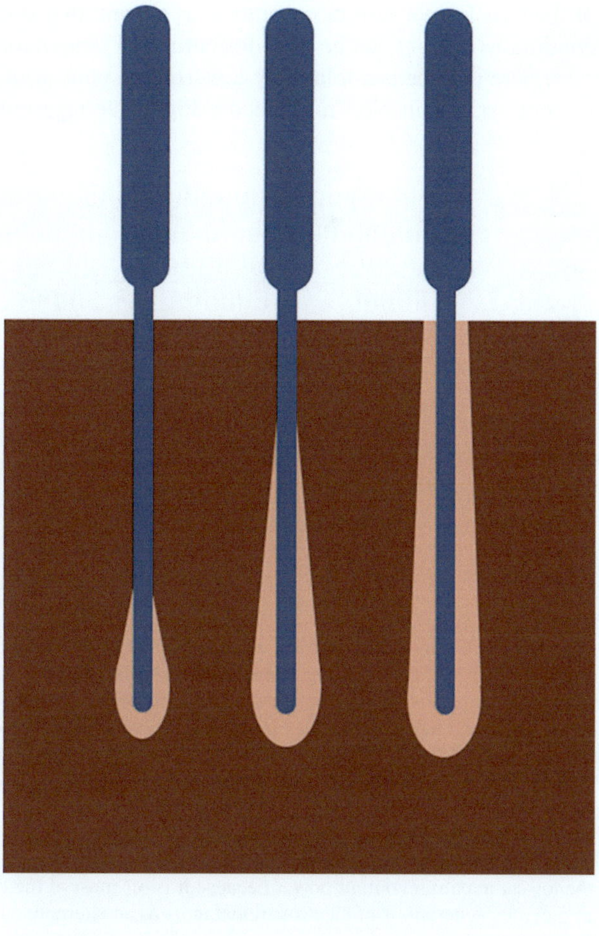

Fig. 3.12 A penetrating needle-shaped active electrode is inserted into the tissue for electrocoagulation. Coagulation starts from the tip of the electrode. With higher energy (continuing current passage for a longer time or using a higher output power), a rim of coagulated tissue forms around the needle in its length; however, this rim is thicker around the tip of the electrode [19, 20]

3.9 Electrosurgical Current Waveforms

Key Points

- Electrosection needs a high-power current. The voltage should be relatively low to avoid large sparks. The cutting mode of electrosurgical devices has a continuous waveform that can provide the maximum output power of the generator at a relatively low voltage.
- Electrofulguration, on the other hand, may need low power. The voltage may need to be relatively high to produce larger sparks. Intermittent currents reduce the output power while keeping the maximum voltage of the current and can be used for a superficial fulguration.

An electrosurgical generator uses household currents to make electrosurgical currents with a variety of waveforms (Fig. 3.13). A transformer inside of the generator takes the input electrical current and increases its frequency and voltage. The output of the transformer will be a continuous current that is called a cutting current. This continuous current can be used for cutting or coagulation.

A pure cut needs a relatively low-voltage current in order to avoid large sparks. In contrast, fulguration may need a higher voltage current to make larger sparks.

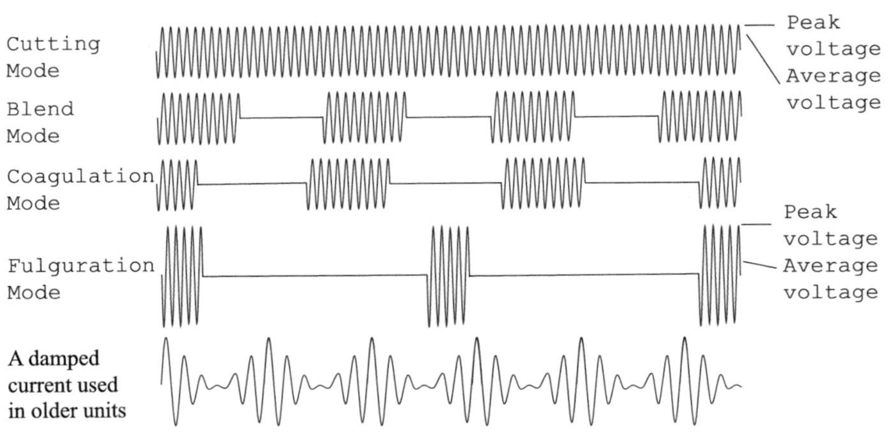

Fig. 3.13 Different electrosurgical current waveforms of a device, each at their maximum output voltage/power settings. Cutting, blend, and coagulation modes of this device originate from the same transformer and have the same maximum peak voltage. Fulguration mode has a different transformer and has a higher maximum peak voltage. Cutting mode uses a continuous waveform which can provide the maximum output power of the generator. Coagulation mode uses the same cutting current and turns it on and off thousands of times per second to make an intermittent waveform. Coagulation mode has a lower maximum power than cutting mode because the delivery of the current is off for some periods of time. Fulguration mode incorporates a higher peak voltage (up to 10,000 volts or higher) which helps with large spark formation. Fulguration mode may have the lowest maximum output power because it is off most of the time. Damped currents were used in previous generations of electrosurgical units as an alternative to interrupted undamped currents

The problem is that a high-voltage continuous current has a high power that is more than what we need for superficial coagulation.

In an attempt to create a high-voltage but low-power current for a superficial fulguration, intermittent currents were created (Fig. 3.13). Intermittent currents turn off and on thousands of times per second; therefore, they look like a continuous current in practice but with lower power than expected for the high voltage. In other words, intermittent currents have a higher ratio of peak-to-average voltage compared with continuous currents.

In an electrosurgical generator, an intermittent current with the same peak voltage as the cutting current may be named blend mode or coagulation mode (Fig. 3.13). This mode must have a lower maximum power output than the continuous cutting mode because it is off sometimes.

If an intermittent current has a higher peak voltage than the cutting mode, it may be named fulguration mode on the front panel of an electrosurgical device (Fig. 3.13).

The name of each waveform or mode (cutting mode, coagulation mode, or fulguration mode) does not necessarily translate to the final effect the mode has on tissue (Table 3.1). A continuous current provided by the cutting mode of an electrosurgical generator can provide coagulation (including fulguration and desiccation), a clean cut, or a blend cut depending on how the current is applied to the tissue. On the other hand, an interrupted current provided by the coagulation or fulguration mode of a generator can provide blend cutting or coagulation but not a pure cut [15].

The variables that determine the final effects of a current on tissue are the rate at which heat is produced, the final temperature, and the depth of the heat. The current waveform, voltage, and power of an electrosurgical current do not have any direct effect on tissue results. However, these parameters can affect the depth and the rate of heat production and indirectly influence the final effect on the tissue [15, 21].

Previous generations of electrosurgical units used spark gaps or vacuum tubes to produce damped intermittent currents with a high ratio of peak-to-average voltage for fulguration. Those damped currents were alternatives for interrupted undamped currents used in newer generations of electrosurgical units and had the same surgical effects. There is a myth in medical literature that damped waveforms provide electrodesiccation and electrofulguration, whereas the application of moderately damped and undamped currents results in electrocoagulation and cutting, respectively. This statement is a misunderstanding that does not have any supporting evidence or scientific explanation. This myth probably originated when the physicians noticed that the damped waveforms were used in the fulguration mode of electrosurgical devices and undamped currents in cutting mode. The fact is that a damped current can provide fulguration, coagulation, or blend cutting, whereas an undamped continuous current can provide all of those mentioned effects plus pure cutting. One should remember that an undamped continuous current may not be the best choice for fulguration.

In an intermittent waveform, the voltage, amperage, and power fluctuate between zero or minimum in the off phases and maximum in the on phases. In this book, we

Table 3.1 Potential uses of different electrosurgical waveforms

Electrosurgical currents (generator mode)	Size of electrode tip	Output power	Potential uses and tissue effects (surgical methods)
Continuous current (cutting mode)	Needle-shaped electrode	Very low power	Superficial contact coagulation. A very low power cannot cut tissues or produce effective fulguration
		Low power	Superficial coagulation. A low power may not be able to cut or produce effective fulguration
		Mid to high power	Cutting if the electrode is pushed into tissue; fulguration if the electrode moves over tissue
	Large-tip electrode	Low power	A low power may not be able to provide enough heating in a large mass of tissue for any surgical effect
		Mid to high power	Fulguration or contact coagulation
Interrupted current (blend cut, coagulation, or fulguration modes)	Needle-shaped electrode	Very low power	Superficial contact coagulation. A very low power cannot cut or produce effective fulguration
		Low power	Superficial contact coagulation or fulguration. A low power may not be able to cut
		Mid to high power	Cutting if the electrode is pushed into tissue; fulguration if the electrode moves over tissue
	Large-tip electrode	Mid to high power	Fulguration or contact coagulation

use the term peak voltage to refer to the maximum voltage of the current during on phases and the terms amperage and power to refer to the mean amperage and mean power of the current.

References

1. Pollack SV. Electrosurgery of the skin, vol. 1. New York: Churchill Livingstone; 1990.
2. Duffy S, Cobb GV. Practical electrosurgery. UK: First. Chapman & Hall. London; 1995.
3. Miklavcic D, Pavcelj N, Hart F. Electric properties of tissues. In: Wiley encyclopedia of biomedical engineering [Internet]. Wiley; 2006. https://doi.org/10.1002/9780471740360.ebs0403.
4. Geddes LA, Baker LE. The specific resistance of biological material – a compendium of data for the biomedical engineer and physiologist. Med Biol Eng. 1967;5(3):271–93. PubMed PMID: 6068939.

5. Christie RV. An experimental study of diathermy: VI. conduction of high frequency currents through the living cell. JExpMed. 1928;48(0022-1007 (Print)):235–46. PubMed PMID: 19869480.
6. Christie RV, Loomis AL. The relation of frequency to the physiological effects of ultra-high frequency currents. JExpMed. 1929;49(0022-1007 (Print)):303–21. PubMed PMID: 19869549.
7. d'Arsonval A. Action physiologique des courants alternatifs a grande frequence. Arch Physiol Norm Path. 1893;5:401–8.
8. Elliott JA. Electrosurgery. Its use in dermatology, with a review of its development and technologic aspects. ArchDermatol. 1966;94(0003-987X (Print)):340–50. PubMed PMID: 4952822.
9. Huntoon RD. Tissue heating accompanying electrosurgery: an experimental investigation. AnnSurg. 1937;105(0003-4932 (Print)):270–90. PubMed PMID: 17856926.
10. Palanker D, Vankov A, Jayaraman P. On mechanisms of interaction in electrosurgery. New J Phys [Internet]. 2008:10. Available from: ISI:000264869500008.
11. Turrell WJ. The physico-chemical action of interrupted currents in relation to their therapeutic effects. ProcRSocMed. 1926;20(0035-9157 (Print)):103–16. PubMed PMID: 19985455.
12. Nernst W, Barratt JOW. Elektrische nervenreizung durch wechselstrome. Zeitschr Elektrochem. 1904;10(35):664–8.
13. Taheri A, Mansoori P, Sandoval LF, Feldman SR, Pearce D, Williford PM. Electrosurgery: Part II. Technology, applications, and safety of electrosurgical devices. J Am Acad Dermatol. 2014;70(4):607.e1-12. https://doi.org/10.1016/j.jaad.2013.09.055. quiz 619–20. PubMed PMID: 24629362.
14. Taheri A, Mansoori P, Huang KE, Feldman SR. Effect of frequency on entrance and propagation pattern of high-frequency (radiofrequency) electrical currents in biologic tissues. Skin Res Technol Off J Int Soc Bioeng Skin ISBS Int Soc Digit Imaging Skin ISDIS Int Soc Skin Imaging ISSI. 2015;21(3):291–4. https://doi.org/10.1111/srt.12191. PubMed PMID: 25329232.
15. Taheri A, Mansoori P, Sandoval LF, Feldman SR, Pearce D, Williford PM. Electrosurgery: Part I. Basics and principles. J Am Acad Dermatol. 2014;70(4):591.e1-14. https://doi.org/10.1016/j.jaad.2013.09.056. quiz 605–6. PubMed PMID: 24629361.
16. Miranda EN. A simple model for understanding the skin effect. Int J Electr Eng Educ. 1999;36(1):31–6. https://doi.org/10.7227/IJEEE.36.1.4.
17. Taheri A, Mansoori P, Bahrami N, Alinia H, Watkins CE, Feldman SR. How frequency of electrosurgical current and electrode size affect the depth of electrocoagulation. Dermatol Surg Off Publ Am Soc Dermatol Surg Al. 2016;42(2):197–202. https://doi.org/10.1097/DSS.0000000000000593. PubMed PMID: 26783688.
18. Krasteva VT, Papazov SP. Estimation of current density distribution under electrodes for external defibrillation. BiomedEng Online. 2002;1(1475-925X (Electronic)):7. PubMed PMID: 12537593.
19. Taheri A, Mansoori P, Feldman SR, Pearce D. High-frequency (radiofrequency) electrical currents entrance and propagation in biological tissues as applied to fractional skin rejuvenation. In: The Orlando Dermatology Aesthetic and Clinical Conference, editor. The Orlando Dermatology Aesthetic and Clinical conference. The Orlando Dermatology Aesthetic and Clinical Conference; 2013.
20. Taheri A, Mansoori P, Sandoval LS, Feldman SR, Williford PM, Pearce D. Entrance and propagation pattern of high-frequency electrical currents in biological tissues as applied to fractional skin rejuvenation using penetrating electrodes. Skin Res Technol. 2013; Online publication ahead of print.
21. Brill AI. Electrosurgery: principles and practice to reduce risk and maximize efficacy. ObstetGynecolClinNorth Am. 2011;38(1558-0474 (Electronic)):687–702. https://doi.org/10.1016/j.ogc.2011.09.005. PubMed PMID: 22134017.

Chapter 4
Basic Mechanism of Electrosurgery

Abstract

- In electrosurgery, a high-frequency alternating electric current flows from the active electrode through the patient's body to the return electrode.
- Adjacent to the active electrode, tissue resistance to the passage of the current converts electrical energy to heat, resulting in thermal tissue damage.
- Current density in tissue rapidly decreases with distance from the active electrode when the current propagates into large masses of tissue under and around the surgical site. Therefore, heat generation is practically confined to the vicinity of the active electrode tip.
- Electrocoagulation occurs when tissue is heated and undergoes thermal denaturation.
- A sudden increase in tissue temperature above boiling point causes rapid explosive vaporization of the water content in the tissue adjacent to the electrode which leads to tissue fragmentation and cutting.
- In this chapter, the term *mode* refers to the generator's output setting selected via the device interface. This selection determines the waveform of the current. The term *method* refers to the actual procedure performed. For example, a coagulation mode delivers an interrupted current, which can be used for performing any method, such as fulguration, contact coagulation, or cutting.

The term electrosurgery refers to the passage of a high-frequency alternating electrical current through the tissue in order to achieve a specific surgical effect, such as cutting or coagulation. Although it is not completely understood exactly how electrosurgery works, heat production and thermal tissue damage caused by tissue resistance to the passage of the electrical current are responsible for at least the majority, if not all, of the tissue effects in electrosurgery [1–6]. In contrast with direct currents or low-frequency currents, high-frequency electrical currents do not cause cell depolarization or neuromuscular excitation.

Each electrosurgical device consists of a high-frequency electrical generator and two electrodes (Fig. 4.1). The electric current flows from the generator to the active electrode, then into the target tissue, then through the patient's body, and then to a large return (dispersive) electrode where current flows back to the electrosurgical generator.

A. Taheri et al., *Advanced Electrosurgery*,
https://doi.org/10.1007/978-3-032-28342-9_4

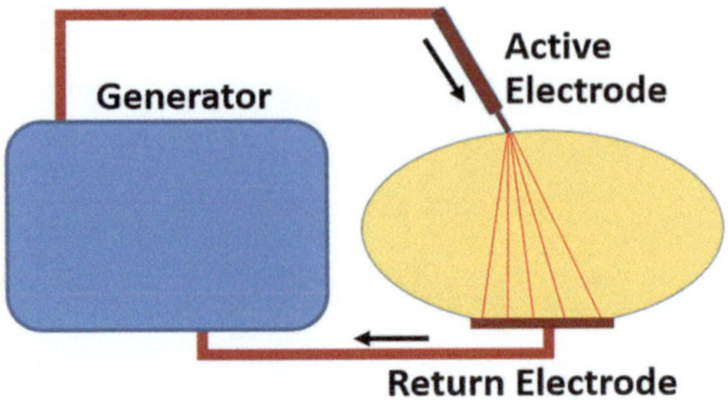

Fig. 4.1 An electrosurgery circuit. An electrosurgical generator provides a high-frequency alternating current. The arrows indicate the direction of the electricity in one phase of the current. In the next phase, the current will be in the opposite direction. The current flows through the tissue, generating heat within the tissue. Heat generation is practically limited to the area of high current density, meaning adjacent to the active electrode

Adjacent to the active electrode, the current is concentrated. Tissue resistance to the passage of this concentrated current converts electrical energy to heat, resulting in thermal tissue damage. Current density in tissue rapidly decreases with distance from the active electrode to a level that cannot induce a significant heating effect. This is the reason the tissue effect of electrosurgery is seen only around the active electrode while the current passes through the deeper tissue as well.

The large return electrode also disperses the current, reducing the current density to levels where tissue heating is minimal.

Electrocoagulation occurs when tissue is heated slowly and undergoes thermal denaturation [2]. Soft tissues usually change their consistency immediately after coagulation. The consistency of the coagulated soft tissues depends on many factors including their water and collagen content. A hydrated epidermis and/or superficial (papillary) dermis turns into a soft doughy material (liquefaction) after coagulation. This soft material can be wiped off the skin using gauze or a blunt curette. In contrast, the deep (reticular) dermis, which has a high concentration of collagen, contracts and turns into a firm tissue immediately after coagulation [7]. Adipocytes or fat cells in subcutaneous fat usually burst upon coagulation. And since there is not much extracellular matrix as structural support between adipocytes, electrosurgery may cut through the adipose tissue even when a relatively low-density current is used with the goal of coagulating.

With continuing the current passage through the coagulated tissue, the temperature increases. This increase in temperature leads to the vaporization of the water content in the coagulated tissue and tissue drying, a process called *desiccation*. A desiccated epidermis has a firm consistency and cannot be wiped off the deeper tissues as easily as a soft coagulated epidermis.

In contrast with coagulation, which happens after a relatively slow increase in tissue temperature, *electrosection* happens after a sudden increase in tissue temperature above the boiling point. If a highly concentrated current passes through a soft tissue, a rapid, explosive vaporization of the water content in the tissue adjacent to the electrode leads to tissue fragmentation, which allows the electrode to pass through the tissue, resulting in cutting [8, 9].

In electrosurgery, heat generation occurs within the tissue, because most metallic cables and electrodes have lower resistivity to electricity than biological tissue. The active electrode acts mainly as a conductor that passes the current and remains cooler than the treated medium. Although the active electrode is not the main source of heat generation, if a relatively high-amperage electrical current passes through a needle-shaped electrode, the electrode may heat up similarly to the target tissue. High temperature in fulguration sparks may also cause heating of a needle-shaped electrode up to its melting point.

4.1 Electrosurgical Methods

An electrosurgical unit can be used for burning (electrocoagulation) or cutting (electrosection) the tissue (Table 4.1).

Table 4.1 Electrosurgical methods and definition of common terms used in electrosurgery

Method	Electrical current or mode of choice	Alternative currents	Definition
Electrocautery	Direct current	Alternating current	An electrical current heats a metallic probe which is then applied to tissue
Electrosurgery	High-frequency alternating current	–	A high-frequency electrical current is passed through the tissue in order to achieve a specific surgical (thermal) effect such as cutting or coagulation
Electrocoagulation (contact coagulation)	Continuous current (cutting mode)[a]	Interrupted currents (blend, coagulation, or fulguration modes)	The tissue is heated below the boiling point and undergoes thermal denaturation
Electrodesiccation	The same as electrocoagulation	The same as electrocoagulation	Vaporization of the water content and drying occurs at superficial tissue layers at the end of coagulation. When desiccation happens, the current cannot pass directly from the active electrode to the tissue in contact mode. At this time, sparks (fulguration) may happen
Electrofulguration (spray or noncontact coagulation)	Interrupted current (fulguration mode)	Interrupted current (coagulation or blend mode) or continuous current (cutting mode)	The active electrode is held above the tissue. The electric current bridges the air gap by creating a spark

(continued)

Table 4.1 (continued)

Method	Electrical current or mode of choice	Alternative currents	Definition
Electrosection, pure cutting	Continuous current (cutting mode)	–	A sudden increase in tissue temperature above boiling point leads to tissue fragmentation and cutting. In pure cutting, there is little coagulation on the incision walls and little hemostasis
Electrosection, blend cutting	Interrupted current (blend or coagulation modes)	–	In blend cutting, there is more coagulation on the incision walls and better hemostasis than pure cutting
Bipolar electrosurgery	Bipolar mode	–	There are two active electrodes. Usually used for coagulation
Monopolar electrosurgery (the opposite of bipolar)	Monopolar modes (cutting, coagulation, desiccation, fulguration)	–	There are one active and one dispersive (return) electrode
Biterminal electrosurgery	–	–	Both active and return electrodes are in contact with the patient's body
Monoterminal electrosurgery (the opposite of biterminal)	–	–	The return electrode is not connected directly to the patient body; instead, it is connected to the earth, and the earth acts as an indirect return electrode

[a]The cutting mode in some electrosurgical units cannot provide a very low power output. In this case, any other mode that can provide a very low power output can be used

4.1.1 Electrocoagulation

Key Points

- Coagulation can be performed in the contact method or the spray (fulguration) method. However, the term electrocoagulation is usually used to refer to coagulation in the contact method.
- At the end of contact electrocoagulation, the more superficial coagulated tissues may dry out (desiccation). The current may decrease or stop flowing at this time, a popping sound may be heard, and sparking may occur through the dried non-conductive layer leading to explosion and fragmentation of the dried layer.
- In contact method, the depth of coagulation is associated with the size of the electrode tip, power, and duration of activation time. A fine-tip electrode is used for superficial electrocoagulation, and a large-tip electrode with a large contact area provides deep coagulation.

- Fulguration mode provides superficial coagulation if a relatively low power is used. It can cause deeper tissue damage if a relatively high power is used, and fulguration continues over a confined area for a longer period.

Electrocoagulation occurs when tissue is heated slowly and undergoes thermal denaturation. The rate at which the tissue temperature rises is proportional to the current density in the tissue. Therefore, a relatively low current density is used for coagulation. A high current density causes a rapid increase in temperature and may lead to tissue explosion and fragmentation or cutting. If a fine-tip electrode is used for coagulation, a very low output power should be selected. A large-tip electrode may need higher output power to provide enough current density for heating and coagulation of a larger area.

Electrocoagulation can be performed in contact method with the electrode kept in contact with the conductive tissue. In this method, the electrode comes in contact with the tissue first. Then the generator is activated. The current passes directly from the electrode into the tissue without any spark or smoke. The tissue in contact with the active electrode should be electrically conductive. A very dry epidermis may not pass the current effectively and may not heat up.

Electrocoagulation may also be performed in spray (fulguration) mode. In this method, the electrosurgical generator is activated first. Then the electrode comes in contact with the tissue. When the electrode contacts the tissue, a very small explosion happens in superficial tissue in contact with the electrode, and sparking forms. Those sparks continue to pass the current through a gap formed of air and smoke between the electrode and the tissue, without any further need for direct contact between the electrode and tissue.

4.1.1.1 Contact Electrocoagulation

For superficial coagulation of small areas (e.g., destruction of small seborrheic keratoses), a fine-tip electrode, such as a needle-shaped electrode or the tip of a knife-shaped electrode, is used. A fine-tip electrode can concentrate a very-low-power current on a small point to provide coagulation. When using a fine-tip electrode, the current density in tissue rapidly decreases with distance from the electrode (Fig. 4.2); therefore, heat generation is practically confined to the vicinity of the electrode tip, potentially decreasing the depth of tissue damage and the possibility of scar formation [10].

When using a large-tip electrode (large electrode–tissue contact surface area) in the contact method, a higher power output should be used to achieve the desired current density and heating in the larger target mass. Current density decreases with distance from the electrode surface more slowly compared with a fine electrode (Fig. 4.2). A higher power output (higher amperage) and slower decrease in current density lead to the presence of a higher current density in deeper layers, resulting in a deeper tissue injury. A large electrode tip (ball- or disk-shaped electrodes or the side of a knife-shaped electrode), therefore, should be used only for deep coagulation, such as the destruction of the deeper dermis after curettage of a malignant skin tumor, if they are used in contact method [11].

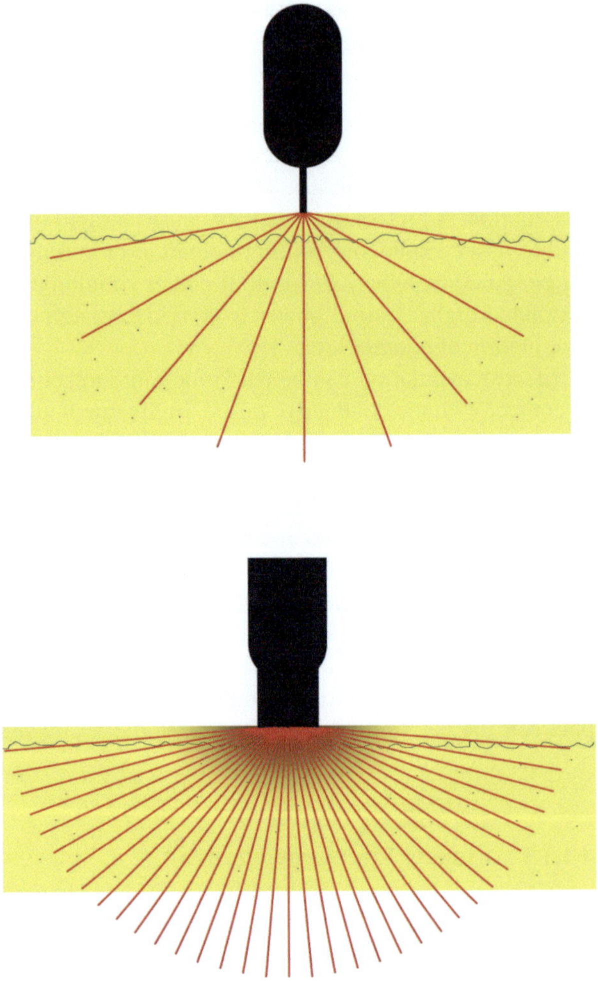

Fig. 4.2 Contact electrocoagulation. A fine electrode needs a low-power setting and is suitable for superficial coagulation. A large-tip electrode is suitable for deep coagulation. A large electrode cannot provide a superficial coagulation because the current density decreases with distance from the electrode surface slowly

Superficial coagulation of large surface areas such as large flat epidermal lesions or hemostasis of large oozing surfaces using a fine-tip electrode in contact method is a slow process and not practical. Spray coagulation or electrofulguration has been developed to speed up superficial coagulation of larger areas.

Electrodesiccation

With continuing contact electrocoagulation, the more superficial tissues may dry out. This stage of coagulation is called desiccation (i.e., drying). This dry layer has a high electrical resistance and decreases or stops the flow of the current, limiting the maximum depth of coagulation (Fig. 4.3). When desiccation happens, a popping

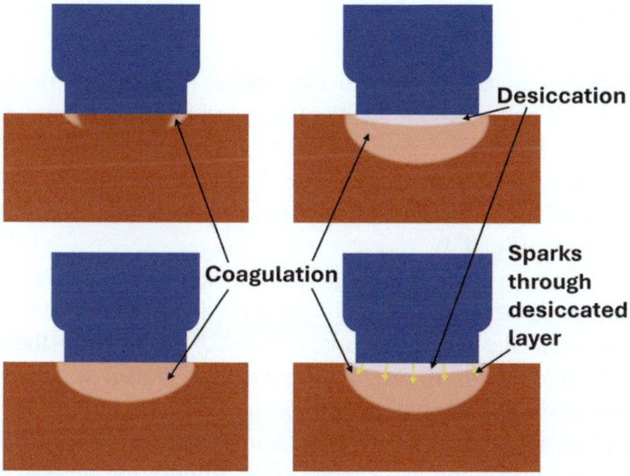

Fig. 4.3 Electrocoagulation and electrodesiccation. At the end of coagulation, the more superficial coagulated tissue dries out (desiccation) and becomes less electrically conductive, potentially preventing the current from continuing to flow (top right). However, sparking may then occur through the nonconductive desiccated layer leading to disruption of this layer, passage of more current, more heat production, and deeper thermal damage (bottom right)

sound may be heard, and/or sparking may occur through the dried nonconductive layer. Those sparks can lead to the explosion and fragmentation of the dried layer. Although fulguration is not a very effective way of providing deep coagulation, if the surgeon continues fulgurating on top of a hot desiccated surface, it may increase the depth of thermal coagulation through heat conduction.

Desiccation is not a method or a distinctive final tissue effect; it is only the final stage of contact coagulation that may or may not happen. It may happen at any time during coagulation regardless of the depth of the coagulated tissue. The timing of the occurrence of desiccation during coagulation depends on the rate of increase in temperature that is the result of current density. With lower current density, there may be a deep coagulation before desiccation happens [2]. Therefore, for a deep coagulation (e.g., after curettage of a malignant skin tumor), a relatively low power should be chosen to provide a slow coagulation and late occurrence of desiccation. However, a very low power may not be able to provide the desired coagulation at all.

Definitions, it seems, have at times hindered a higher level of understanding of electrosurgery. The term electrodesiccation has been used in literature as a distinctive method from coagulation. Some authors use the term electrodesiccation to refer to monoterminal electrocoagulation while reserving the term electrocoagulation to refer to biterminal electrocoagulation [12–14]. Others use the term electrodesiccation to refer to contact electrocoagulation as opposed to spray electrocoagulation (fulguration) [6, 15]. Although tissue drying also occurs during fulguration, the term electrodesiccation is mainly used to refer to the final stage of contact coagulation.

4.1.1.2 Electrofulguration

In electrofulguration, an activated electrode touches the tissue while the generator is activated. The first touch between the electrode and the tissue starts an electric discharge arc (spark). Then the active electrode is held above the tissue. Using the high-voltage current, the gap of air between the electrode and the tissue is bridged by a spark. The spark rapidly dances from one spot to the other, reestablishing itself at different locations (Fig. 4.4).

When using a fine-tip electrode, large dancing sparks spread the current over an area larger than the tip of the electrode like a spray [16]. The higher the voltage, the larger the sparks, and the larger the spray "brush." By moving the electrode and spraying the current over tissue, coagulation can be achieved on a large surface area faster than when operating in contact with tissue.

A large-tip electrode such as a ball-shaped or flat side of a knife-shaped electrode can act like a larger brush and can speed up the fulguration process by covering a larger surface area with each pass of the electrode on tissue than a fine-tip electrode (Fig. 4.5). A large-tip electrode may not need a high-voltage fulguration current to work fast.

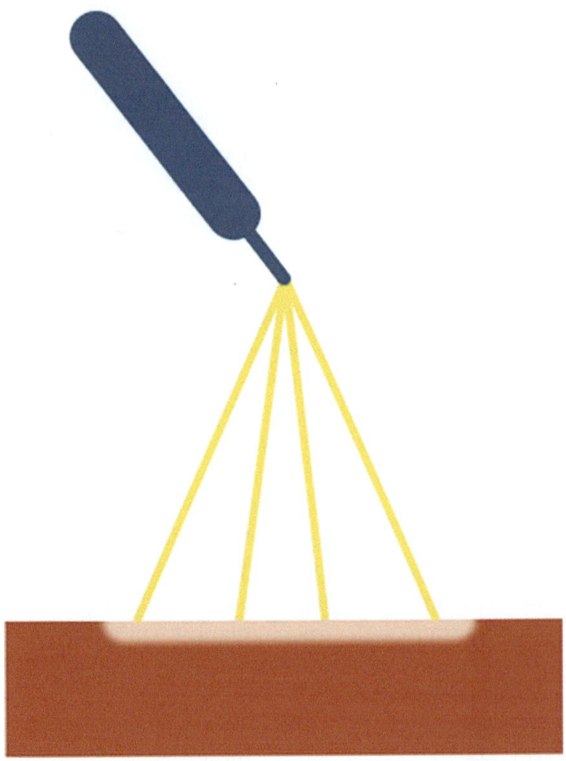

Fig. 4.4 Fulguration using a fine-tip electrode. Large dancing sparks spread the current over an area larger than the tip of the electrode

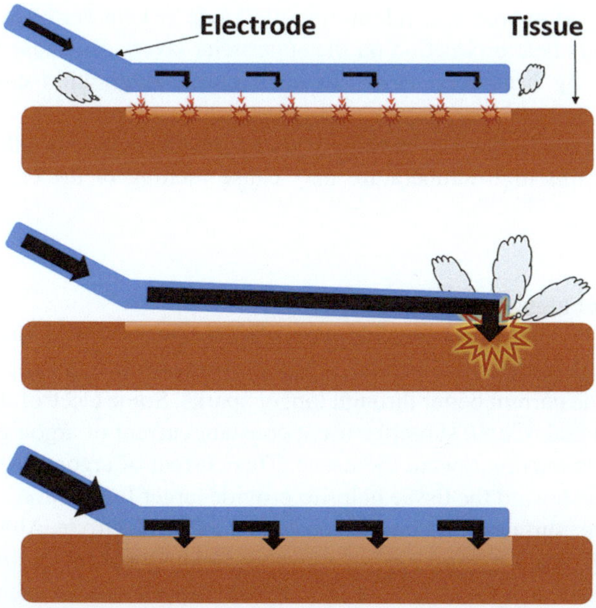

Fig. 4.5 Top: A large-tip electrode is used in fulguration mode. The surgeon is applying enough pressure to keep the electrode in good "contact" with the tissue. However, there is no direct physical contact between the electrode and the tissue. Sparks pass a relatively low-power current through the high resistance gap between the electrode and the tissue. The gas produced from tissue explosion at the end of the sparks keeps the gap and prevents the electrode from touching the tissue. Middle: If a part of the electrode comes in direct contact with the tissue, the circuit resistance falls, and a higher current will be concentrated on that spot causing tissue explosion. This explosion pushes the electrode away from the tissue again restarting fulguration. Bottom: If a large part of the electrode comes in contact with the tissue, or if the power output is relatively low, no explosion may occur. With no explosion or spark, coagulation will continue in the contact method. The current increases because of relatively low resistance at the electrode–tissue interface. The new contact method may cause a deeper coagulation than the fulguration method

During electrofulguration, the active electrode may come in contact with the tissue. If the electrode touches the tissue at any point, the current will be concentrated on that spot, causing tissue explosion. This explosion and the resulting hot gas push the electrode away from the tissue, returning it to the fulguration mode (Fig. 4.5). However, if a large part of the electrode comes in contact with the tissue or if the output power is not enough for tissue explosion, the electrode may stick to the tissue. If it happens, no sparks can be seen or heard, and fulguration will change to contact coagulation (Fig. 4.5).

In electrofulguration, each spark carries the current to a very small point at a moment, acting as a very fine electrode. At the end of each spark, the temperature is extremely high, leading to tissue explosion and fragmentation or charring. If a relatively low power is used, current density and temperature drop rapidly with distance from the end of the sparks, and thermal damage will be limited to a thin superficial layer of tissue. However, if a fulgurating electrode is kept active over a confined area, continuous heat production on the superficial layers can cause the heating of deeper layers by heat conduction. In such cases, fulguration can cause deep coagulation.

Fulguration sparks have an extremely high temperature. If a needle-shaped electrode is used, this high temperature may cause melting of the end of the active electrode.

Argon Plasma Fulguration

When put in an electromagnetic field, argon gas turns to plasma more easily than air and can pass the current better through longer sparks. Some electrofulguration electrodes used in endoscopic surgeries use a constant current of argon gas around the active electrode moving toward the tissue. This current of argon traveling from the active electrode toward the tissue helps to provide larger fulguration sparks in order to cover a larger surface of tissue with each pass of the electrode. Although the final tissue effect of argon fulguration is similar to conventional fulguration, the procedure can be done faster with a more homogenous application of the current on the target, when the sparks travel in argon. This method can be used for hemostasis of bleeding surfaces. In dermatologic surgery, using a larger-tip electrode is easy and eliminates any need for argon plasma.

4.1.1.3 Factors Influencing the Depth of Coagulation

The depth of coagulation depends on the amount of heat generation (output power multiplied by activation time) per surface unit of tissue, as well as the depth at which heat is generated (Table 4.2).

In the fulguration method, heat generation is in superficial tissue. If a low output power is used and the electrode moves fast on the tissue (short activation time), tissue damage is superficial. However, if the electrode moves slowly on tissue while using a high output power, more heat generation leads to more heat conduction to the deeper tissue resulting in deeper damage at the cost of significant smoke formation.

In the contact method, a fine-tip electrode can confine heat generation to the superficial layer of the tissue (Fig. 4.2). Using a very low output power and a short activation time, coagulation will be superficial. Using a high output power with a fine-tip electrode provides a very high concentration of current in a small area causing tissue explosion. This tissue explosion changes contact coagulation to fulguration (if the electrode is kept on top of the tissue) or cutting (if the electrode is pushed into the tissue).

A large-tip electrode in contact mode needs a relatively high output power and delivers a higher current density into deeper layers, resulting in a deeper tissue injury (Fig. 4.2). When using a large-tip electrode, the coagulation at the

Table 4.2 Settings of electrosurgical units based on the desired depth of coagulation

Depth of tissue injury	Area	Method of application of current	Electrical current or mode of choice	Alternative currents	Setting	Possible indications
Superficial destruction	Small area	Fine-tip electrode and contact method	Continuous current (cutting mode)	Interrupted current (blend or coagulation modes)	Usually, a very-low-power setting is used. The power is started very low and is increased until a reasonably fast movement of the electrode on the target can be attained. Coagulated materials can be wiped off and a second pass may be performed if necessary	Ablation of epidermis and papillary dermis Small seborrheic keratosis Lentigo Syringoma Cherry angioma Spider angioma Sebaceous hyperplasia
	Large area	Fine- or large-tip electrode and fulguration[a] method	Interrupted current (fulguration mode)	Interrupted current (coagulation mode). If using a large-tip electrode, cutting mode can also be used	Depending on the speed of movement of the electrode, a low- to medium-power setting is used. The power is started low and is increased until a reasonably fast movement of the electrode on the target can be attained	Seborrheic keratosis Verrucous epidermal nevus Hemostasis

(continued)

Table 4.2 (continued)

Depth of tissue injury	Area	Method of application of current	Electrical current or mode of choice	Alternative currents	Setting	Possible indications
Medium depth destruction	Small to large area	Medium-size-tip electrode and contact method or fine- or large-tip electrode and fulguration method	Depending on the method (see above)	Depending on the method	Needs more power than superficial destruction. If curettage or shaving is performed before electrosurgery, achievement of hemostasis using electrosurgery can be (but is not necessarily) an indicator of the adequacy of treatment. Multiple passes or slow movement of the electrode on the tissue can provide deeper coagulation	Rhinophyma Bowen's disease Low-risk basal cell carcinoma[b] Pyogenic granuloma[b]
Deep destruction (usually used as an alternative to excision)	Medium to large area	Large-tip electrode and contact method	Continuous current (cutting mode)	Interrupted currents (blend or coagulation modes)	Medium- to high-power setting. The power should be enough for a slow desiccation (hearing a popping sound after a few seconds). The slower the desiccation process, the deeper the damage	Basal cell carcinoma[b] Keratoacanthoma[b] Squamous cell carcinoma[b]

[a]Depending on the power and the speed of movement of the electrode on the target, electrofulguration potentially can induce either a very superficial or a relatively deep destruction

[b]Friable tumors can be treated using curettage and electrocoagulation as an alternative to excision

electrode–tissue interface may not be homogenous. The coagulation may start along the perimeter and extremities of the electrode–tissue contact area and may go deep before the tissue in contact with the center of the electrode coagulates.

One may propose that choosing a low-power setting and a longer activation time for contact coagulation can be safer and produce the same result as choosing a higher power and a shorter activation time. However, this is not the case. Longer activation time results in more heat conduction and collateral tissue damage before the desired outcome is attained [17, 18]. This is similar to choosing the pulse duration of lasers. Therefore, in order to minimize the collateral tissue damage (e.g., during the destruction of flat seborrheic keratoses), the activation time should be short or divided into multiple pulses separated by periods of time long enough to allow the tissue to cool before the next pulse.

4.1.2 Electrosection

Key Points

- For a pure cutting with a relatively clean incision and little hemostasis, a thin needle-shaped electrode and a continuous cutting current (cut mode) are used. The cutting of the tissue should be brisk with the lowest possible power setting.
- A thick electrode cannot provide a pure clean cut.
- Blend cutting provides a thicker layer of coagulation on the incision walls and better hemostasis than pure cutting. It can be performed using an interrupted current (blend or coagulation mode).

Electrosection provides a means of cutting tissue in place of a scalpel. The major advantage of this method of cutting is that hemostasis is achieved immediately upon incision by coagulation on either side of the incision wall. Larger blood vessels may still require additional spot coagulation after the cutting to achieve hemostasis.

A thin needle or wire electrode can concentrate a relatively lower-power current on a small area in its vicinity, providing a very high current density that can lead to tissue explosion and cutting. Like a fine-tip coagulation electrode, the current density and heat generation in tissue rapidly decrease with distance from the electrode (Fig. 4.6). By limiting heat generation to its vicinity, a needle can limit the depth of coagulation on the incision walls. Therefore, a thin needle or wire is used to make a relatively clean incision with minimal coagulation and hemostasis (Fig. 4.6).

A thick needle electrode can cut through the tissue if a relatively high-power current is used. In this case, similar to a large-tip coagulation electrode (Fig. 4.2), current density and temperature decrease with distance from the electrode more slowly compared with a thin electrode (Fig. 4.6) [10]. The result is a deeper coagulation margin on incision walls during cutting that leads to more effective hemostasis. This mode is called blend cut, meaning a blend of cutting and coagulation (Fig. 4.6).

When the cutting electrode comes in contact with the tissue, an initial tissue heating and explosive vaporization of the medium around the electrode leads to the

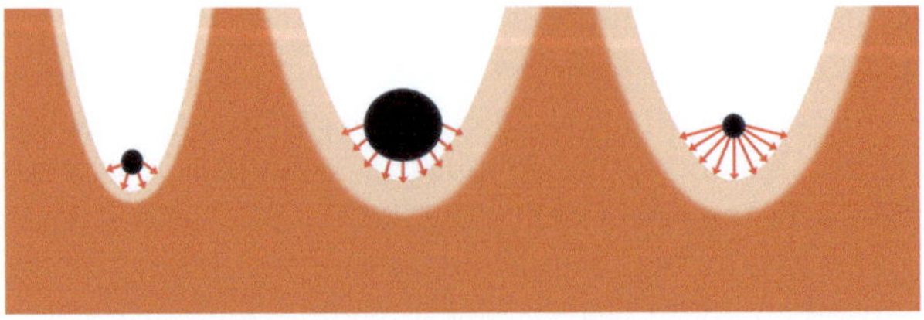

Fig. 4.6 Cross section of tissue treated with three cutting electrodes. Left: A thin needle can concentrate a low-peak-voltage low-power current (cutting current with relatively low power) on a small area and make a relatively clean incision with little coagulation on the incision walls. Middle: A thick electrode can cut through the tissue if a higher-power current is used. The result is deeper coagulation margins. Right: A high-peak-voltage current (blend or coagulation waveforms) produces large sparks and acts as if a thicker electrode is being used that cannot concentrate the current

isolation of the metallic electrode from the tissue. Ionization of the vapor around the electrode allows maintaining the current through the vapor cavity by sparks, similar to fulguration. Therefore, the cutting may continue without direct contact between the active electrode and the tissue [10]. The higher the peak voltage of the current (e.g., fulguration mode), the larger the sparks (Fig. 4.6). Larger sparks can spread current to a wider area of tissue around the electrode and act as if a thicker electrode is being used that cannot concentrate the current in a small area [19]. Therefore, an interrupted high-peak-voltage current provides deeper collateral tissue coagulation on either side of the incision walls and better hemostasis (Fig. 4.6) [2, 20]. Blend mode or coagulation mode currents of electrosurgical generators are interrupted and have a higher ratio of peak to average voltage than pure cut currents and can be used for making a blend cut. Depending on the technique used, the depth of coagulation on either side of an electrosurgical incision varies from 0.1 to 2 mm [21–23]. Fulguration mode has the lowest power output compared with the other modes in most generators and may not be able to provide enough current for cutting. However, if fulguration mode is used for cutting, it produces a very thick coagulation on the incision walls, because of its very high ratio of peak to average voltage.

In order to have a pure cut with less collateral tissue damage and coagulation on the incision walls, like electrocoagulation, contact time should be reduced to minimize heat production and conduction [17]. Therefore, the cutting of the tissue should be brisk with the lowest effective power setting [9]. When the power setting is too low, the cutting process may be slow, resulting in wider collateral coagulation [24]. The correct output power for a clean incision can be determined by starting low and increasing the power until the maximum cutting speed can be attained. If the power is insufficient, the electrode does not glide through the tissue easily, essentially "sticking" [6]. If large arcing or sparking is seen across the tissue surface, voltage is too high and should be appropriately reduced.

By providing some hemostasis, electrosection can significantly reduce surgical time and blood loss during surgery [25]. Although there are some concerns regarding the use of electrosection when primary closure of the surgical wound is planned, previous studies have not shown any significant difference in wound infection rates or scar cosmesis between surgical wounds created with electrosection versus traditional scalpel surgery.

If a needle-shaped cutting electrode is used, extremely high temperatures caused by sparks may cause the melting of the electrode. The manufacturers use metals with very high melting temperatures such as tungsten for making needle-shaped electrodes to reduce the risk of melting.

4.2 Bipolar Versus Monopolar Electrosurgery

Key Points

- In monopolar electrosurgery, there is an active electrode and a dispersive electrode, while in bipolar mode, there are two active electrodes.
- In bipolar mode, electrical current passes only through the tissue grasped between the tips of the bipolar forceps; therefore, this mode may be potentially safer than monopolar mode.

In electrosurgery, the prefixes "mono-" and "bi-" polar refer to the number of active electrodes. In monopolar electrosurgery, an active electrode carries current to the tissue (Fig. 4.1). Current then spreads through the body to be collected and returned to the electrosurgery unit by a large-surface dispersive electrode. The dispersive electrode is also known as the return, neutral, passive, or patient plate electrode.

Two types of dispersive electrodes are in common use today, the conductive type and the capacitive type. With the conductive type, a metallic foil or conductive polymer is attached to the patient's skin. With the capacitive type, the conductive foil has an insulating layer on the outside that prevents direct contact with the patient's skin. The insulated electrode and the patient's skin form a capacitor that passes a capacitive current. Both types of dispersive electrodes have specific advantages and disadvantages. Electrode failures and subsequent patient injury can be attributed mostly to improper application, electrode dislodgment, and electrode defects rather than to electrode design [16].

Monopolar electrosurgery should be performed with caution on an extremity such as a finger or penis because there is limited cross-sectional area for the return current to spread across. Theoretically, this may result in higher current density and some heating throughout the volume of the extremity leading to unintentional thermal damage. Very-low-power electrosurgery is generally safe on fingers. If a medium-power output is used, the activation time should be short. In order to reduce the risk even more, the target finger can be wrapped to adjacent fingers using a gauze soaked in saline to increase the cross-sectional area for the return current to spread across. Achieving deep electrocoagulation on a relatively large area needs a lot of power and heat production and is generally not recommended on a finger or penis.

Unlike monopolar electrosurgery where the patient's body forms a major part of the electrical circuit, in bipolar electrosurgery, only the tissue grasped between the

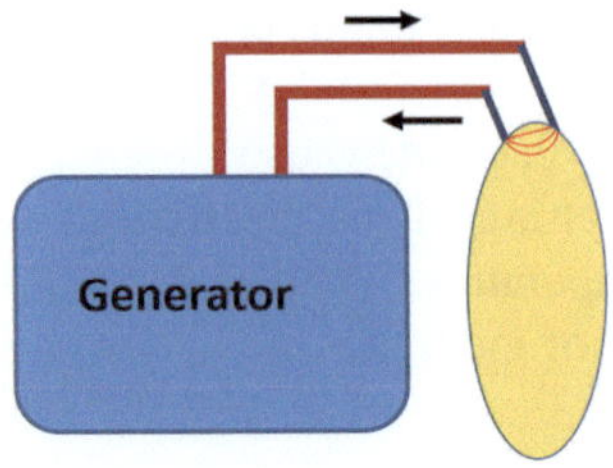

Fig. 4.7 Bipolar electrosurgery circuit. The electric current flows from one forceps tine, through the tissue placed between the tips, to the other forceps tine, and then back to the electrosurgical generator. Bipolar mode is safer than monopolar mode regarding the potential extent of injury and the possibility of distant site burns

tips of a bipolar forceps is included in the electrical circuit (Fig. 4.7). These bipolar forceps act as two active electrodes.

The bipolar mode is used primarily for coagulation of pedunculated benign tumors or hemostasis of blood vessels. It potentially causes less damage to the surrounding tissue and reduces some of the risks to the patient compared to monopolar electrosurgery. Bipolar mode is safer than monopolar mode on extremities like penis and also for patients that have implanted electronic devices.

4.3 Biterminal Versus Monoterminal Electrosurgery

Key Points

- If electrosurgery is performed with no dispersive electrode connected to the patient's body, the method is called monoterminal electrosurgery. Monoterminal mode can only be performed using *earth-referenced* electrosurgical units that have a return electrode connected to the earth. In this technique, the earth acts as the return electrode.
- In *isolated* electrosurgical units, the return electrode is not connected to the earth. Therefore, there will be no current flow and no thermal effect unless the dispersive electrode is attached to the patient's body (biterminal mode).
- Biterminal mode has a higher maximum power and can be potentially a safer method than monoterminal mode.
- Coagulation, fulguration, and electrosection can be performed in either biterminal or monoterminal mode; however, biterminal mode is the preferred mode for electrosection.

The prefix "mono-" and "bi-" terminal refers to the number of electrodes (active ± return electrode) that are in contact with the patient's body (Figs. 4.1 and 4.8). If both active and return electrodes are connected to the patient body, the method is called biterminal. In the monoterminal method, the surgeon uses only the active electrode, while the return electrode is not connected to the patient.

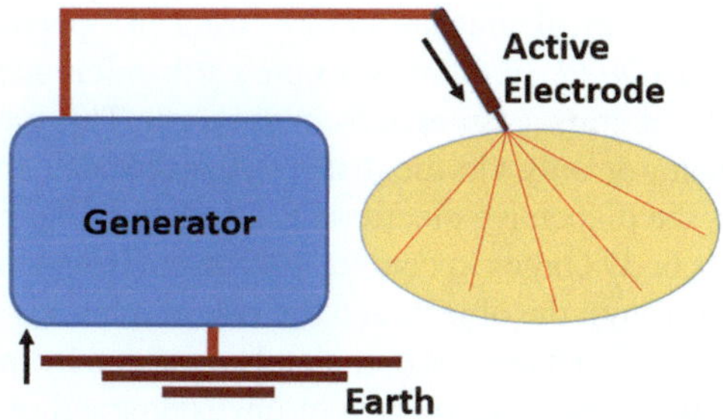

Fig. 4.8 Monoterminal electrosurgery using an earth-referenced unit. The return electrode is connected to the earth. Therefore, the earth and all conductive objects around the patient's body can act as a capacitive-type return electrode. The current passes through the earth and comes back to the generator

In so-called "earth-referenced" electrosurgical units, the return electrode is connected to the earth (usually through the power supply cable), and therefore the earth and all conductive objects around the patient's body can act as a capacitive-type dispersive electrode (Fig. 4.8). Performing monopolar electrosurgery without using a dispersive electrode is called monoterminal or single-electrode electrosurgery (Fig. 4.8). Because the maximum output power is far lower when the dispersive electrode is not used, only relatively low-powered electrosurgery can be performed in monoterminal mode. Monoterminal mode reduces the power but not the peak voltage; therefore, a pure cut cannot be performed using this mode. This is the reason biterminal electrosurgery is the preferred mode for electrosection. On the other hand, by reducing the power but not the peak voltage, the monoterminal method can provide larger, low-powered sparks that can be a good choice for fulguration when the plan is superficial coagulation of a large surface area using a fine-tip electrode.

There is a risk of burning at nonsurgical sites when the return electrode is not in use. During monoterminal electrosurgery with an earth-referenced unit, if an electrically conductive object such as a metal table, electrocardiogram electrode, or surgical staff comes into contact with the patient's body, some current may select the object as a low-resistance return pathway to the ground. If the contact area is small, the current concentration at this point may result in a burn at this site. For this reason, monoterminal mode is used only on conscious patients who would be aware of such complications and only on carefully insulated tables. Using a good return electrode ensures that the current returns to the path of least resistance and does not take any alternative path through operators or environmental objects. Therefore, the use of the return electrode, although not technically necessary for the operation of an earth-referenced unit, will enhance the power and potential safety of the electrosurgical apparatus. Earth-referenced electrosurgical units are not commonly used in operating rooms today. However, many surgeons prefer them for outpatient, office-based minor surgical procedures, because of their convenience and for avoiding the additional time and cost associated with the use of a dispersive electrode.

The type of electrosurgical unit commonly used in operating rooms today is known as *floating* or *isolated*. In contrast to the earth-referenced units, the dispersive electrode of isolated units is isolated from the earth. This means that the current can return to the generator only via the dispersive electrode. An isolated generator will not work unless the dispersive electrode is attached to the patient. During activation, if the patient's body comes in contact with an environmental object, very low or no current passes through the object, and the risk of a burn is low. Unfortunately, a high-frequency current is not always completely confined by insulation, and therefore the isolation of these units from earth or environmental objects is never complete. Current leakage does occur by forming a capacitor between electrode cables and the floor of the operating room or conductive environmental objects [26]. And, therefore, there is still a potential for burn at nonsurgical sites if the patient's body comes in contact with metal environmental objects.

When using an earth-referenced generator, if the surgeon touches an activated surgical electrode, he or she may burn. When using an isolated unit, the surgeon may burn herself or himself only if he or she touches the patient (which is connected to the return electrode) with the other hand.

Although a good dispersive electrode reduces the risk of distant site burns, inadequate contact of the dispersive electrode with the patient's body may result in a smaller contact area that concentrates the current and may lead to a burn at that site. Most modern isolated electrosurgery units include a contact quality monitor for the dispersive electrode which measures the quality of the contact between the patient's skin and the dispersive electrode and also between the electrode and the generator (Fig. 4.9). If the dispersive electrode becomes dislodged or there is a high resistance between the dispersive electrode and the patient's skin, the unit will sound an alarm and the power will be disabled. Although, theoretically, this technology reduces the risk of burns at the dispersive electrode site, there is no strong study or clinical evidence supporting this idea. There also have not been any clinical trials comparing

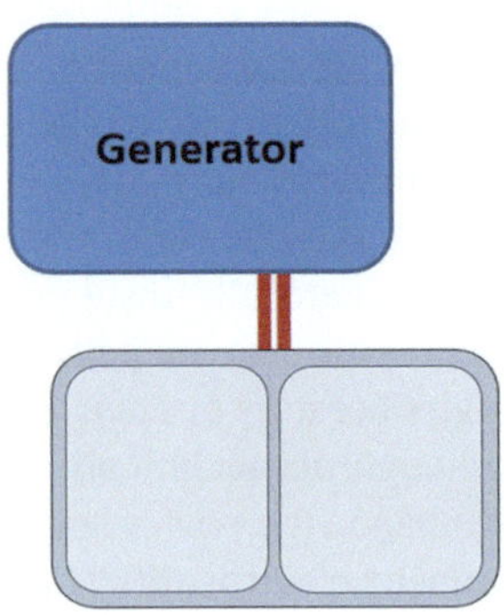

Fig. 4.9 An electrosurgery unit with a contact quality monitor for the dispersive electrode. Contact quality is monitored by splitting the return electrode into two parts and measuring the resistance between the parts. If both parts are in good contact with the skin, the resistance between them will be low. If one or both parts are not in good contact with the skin, the resistance will be high, and the monitoring system will disable the power

the rate of side effects between an earth reference monoterminal device and a biterminal isolated device with or without a contact quality monitor.

The best location for placement of the dispersive electrode is a muscular site well supplied with blood vessels and adjacent to the surgical field. If there is any metal or implanted electronic device in the patient's body, the dispersive pad should be placed between the metal and the surgical site to prevent current from passing selectively through the metal.

4.4 Controlling the Output Power of Electrosurgical Devices

Key Points

- In most electrosurgical generators, voltage is the output variable that can be adjusted on the display panel. The power deployed in tissue is not only dependent on this voltage but also on the resistance in the circuit which is mainly at the electrode–tissue contact area.
- In some devices, power is the output variable that is adjusted on the display panel. In these devices, an *automatic power adjustment* system provides a constant output power regardless of tissue resistance. These devices are rarely if ever used in dermatologic surgery.

There are two types of electrosurgical generators regarding the output-power control system: *constant-voltage* and *automatic power adjustment* [16, 27].

Constant-Voltage Output Systems

Most conventional electrosurgical generators use a *constant-voltage output* system. In these generators, voltage is the output variable that can be adjusted on the display panel. The dial setting for control of voltage in older units is usually calibrated using numbers from 1 to 10. With increasing this number (1–10), the voltage increases as well as the maximum power output that can be delivered. In other words, setting 1 has lower voltage and lower maximum power output than setting 2. One should bear in mind that the actual power deployed in the tissue depends not only on the voltage but also on the resistance in the circuit which is dependent on the quality and size of tissue in contact with the active electrode. These generators deliver less power to the tissue with higher resistance compared to the tissue with lower resistance ($W = V^2/R$, where W = power, V = voltage, and R = resistance) [16, 27]. Therefore, working on a dried hyperkeratotic epidermis may need a higher voltage to be dialed than when working on well-hydrated tissues.

When working with a constant-voltage conventional electrosurgical unit, if a larger part of the active electrode comes in contact with tissue (larger contact area between active electrode and tissue), resistance falls. This allows higher power to be deployed which is necessary for a large electrode to work on a large target (Fig. 4.10). Therefore, the surgeon does not need to dial up the voltage when using a larger part of the active electrode. However, each setting has a maximum output power

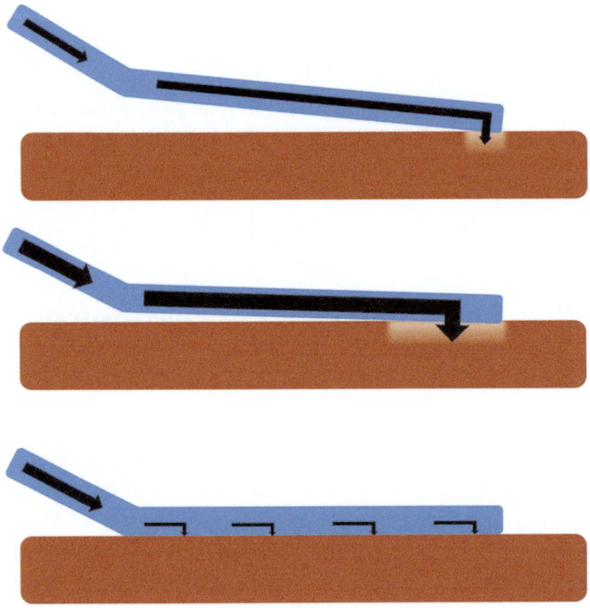

Fig. 4.10 A constant-voltage electrosurgical unit. Top: A surgeon is using the tip of a knife-shaped electrode with a relatively low-power setting. Middle: The surgeon increases the size of the contact area by pressing a larger part of the electrode against the tissue. Resistance in the circuit falls, and a higher-amperage current (more power) flows that provides enough power for working on a larger target. This is an advantage of constant-voltage output systems over automatic power adjustment systems because automatic power adjustment systems cannot increase the power in response to changes in the size of the electrode. Bottom: The surgeon uses a much larger part of the knife. The resistance in the circuit falls too low (below the nominal resistance of the generator). Therefore, the output power of the generator drops. The current density in tissue drops even more. In other words, there is not enough power to heat the large target in contact with the electrode. Although this is a limitation of using constant-voltage output systems, it is an even bigger problem when using automatic power adjustment systems

(Figs. 4.10 and 4.11). A very low voltage (low maximum power) setting dialed on a unit may be enough only for a small electrode. If a very large active electrode is used, that low voltage setting may not be able to provide enough power to induce any surgical effect (Figs. 4.10 and 4.11). In this case, the surgeon can choose a higher maximum output power by increasing the voltage on the control panel of the device or switching to a continuous waveform (cutting mode) that has a higher maximum power.

More recent constant-voltage generators are supplemented with an arbitrary dial setting with a display calibrated in watts. This indicated power refers to the *maximum* power that can be delivered to a nominal resistance in the circuit (Fig. 4.12). A resistance in the circuit that is higher or lower than the nominal resistance leads to an output power lower than the maximum power. Therefore, the power that is

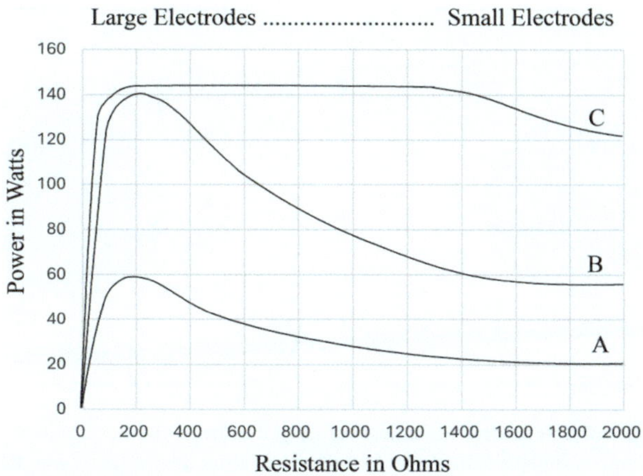

Fig. 4.11 Power-resistance curves of an electrosurgical unit. Each setting has a maximum output power that can be delivered in the case of an ideal resistance (nominal resistance or nominal load) in the circuit. If a very large active electrode is used, a very large contact area leads to a resistance lower than the nominal resistance in the circuit, resulting in reduced output power which may lead to the inability to achieve the desired surgical effect. (**a**) Constant-voltage mode with a nominal load of 200 ohms, when the maximum power is set at 60 watts. (**b**) The same mode when the maximum power is set at 140 watts. Increasing the size of the electrode leads to lower resistance and higher power. Therefore, the current density at the electrode–tissue interface and quality of tissue effect (except for the depth of effect) will not change significantly with changing the size of the electrode. However, a very large electrode–tissue contact area with less than 200 ohms resistance leads to a reduction in power. (**c**) Automatic power adjustment mode provides a constant output power between 200 and 1400 ohms. This unit does not automatically adjust the power according to the electrode size between 200 and 1400 ohms

delivered to the tissue is usually lower than the *maximum* that is dialed on the control panel. This type of display has the advantage of allowing a limited degree of comparison to be made between different units or modes.

Automatic Power Adjustment System

In electrosurgical generators with an automatic power adjustment system (tissue-responsive or tissue-adaptive generators), power is the output variable that can be adjusted on the display panel with the dial setting calibrated in watts. These generators can provide constant power in a wide range of resistances in the circuit (Fig. 4.11c). They can provide the same surgical effect in different tissues with different electrical resistances, at the same power setting [16, 27]. However, if the electrode–tissue contact area increases, power does not increase in proportion to the contact area. Therefore, the power setting should be increased manually to provide enough power to warm up a larger area and create the same surgical effect. Although this is not an issue in endoscopic surgeries where the size of active electrodes may not change, it is a limitation of these generators for use in dermatologic surgeries

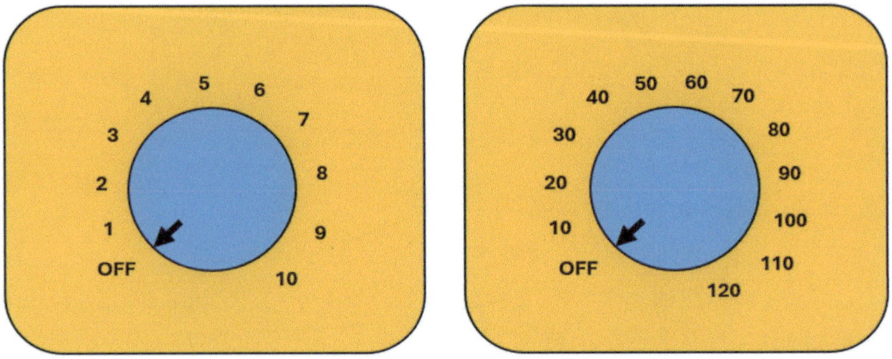

Fig. 4.12 Front-panel dial setting for adjusting output voltage (and consequently power) in two models of a constant-voltage electrosurgical unit. Both units have exactly the same internal parts and have the same maximum power output of 120 watts. The only difference between the units is the numbers printed on the front panel. Left: The dial setting in the older model is calibrated using numbers from 1 to 10. When dialed to 10, the output voltage will be maximum. If there is an ideal (nominal) resistance in the circuit, the maximum power of 120 watts can be delivered. Right: A more recent version of the same generator supplemented with an arbitrary dial setting with a display calibrated in watts. Again, this dial system controls directly the voltage, not the power. This indicated power refers to the maximum power that can be delivered to a nominal resistance in the circuit on that setting. Newer versions of electrosurgical units have digital dial systems with the ability to fine-tune the voltage and power easier especially at very-low-power settings

where the surgeons may need to change the size of the electrode–tissue interface frequently. Although most dermatologic surgeons may prefer constant-voltage generators for their lower price and ease of use, both technologies have specific advantages and disadvantages.

Smart Power Adjustment for Bipolar Hemostasis and Vessel Sealing
Bipolar electrosurgery is widely used for hemostasis of bleeding vessels, especially in endoscopic surgeries. During the procedure, the tissue between the tips of the forceps heats up and coagulates, leading to the sealing of the vessel. With the continuing flow of current, the coagulated tissue desiccates. At the time of desiccation, sparking, fulguration, and explosion of the tissue may happen, which makes the coagulated tissue unstable for maintaining hemostasis. To avoid tissue explosion, the surgeon may stop the current flow when they hear a boiling or popping sound (popping sound implies the start of desiccation) during the procedure.

Some electrosurgical devices use smart power adjustment for bipolar hemostasis and vessel sealing. When coagulation of the tissue is complete and desiccation starts to happen, there is an increase in tissue resistance to the current. These smart systems sense this increase in resistance between the tips of the forceps after coagulation and stop the current just before complete desiccation [27].

References

1. Wang K, Advincula AP. "Current thoughts" in electrosurgery. Int J Gynaecol Obstet. 2007;97(0020-7292 (Print)):245–50. https://doi.org/10.1016/j.ijgo.2007.03.001. PubMed PMID: 17451712.
2. Brill AI. Electrosurgery: principles and practice to reduce risk and maximize efficacy. Obstet Gynecol Clin N Am. 2011;38(1558-0474 (Electronic)):687–702. https://doi.org/10.1016/j.ogc.2011.09.005. PubMed PMID: 22134017.
3. Christie RV, Binger CA. An experimental study of diathermy: iv. Evidence for the penetration of high frequency currents through the living body. J Exp Med. 1927;46(0022-1007 (Print)):715–34. PubMed PMID: 19869368.
4. Finelli A, Rewcastle JC, Jewett MA. Cryotherapy and radiofrequency ablation: pathophysiologic basis and laboratory studies. Curr Opin Urol. 2003;13(0963-0643 (Print)):187–91. https://doi.org/10.1097/01.mou.0000068743.82465.25. PubMed PMID: 12692439.
5. Solbiati L, Ierace T, Goldberg SN, Sironi S, Livraghi T, Fiocca R, et al. Percutaneous US-guided radio-frequency tissue ablation of liver metastases: treatment and follow-up in 16 patients. Radiology. 1997;202(0033-8419 (Print)):195–203. PubMed PMID: 8988211.
6. Van Way CW, Hinrichs CS. Electrosurgery 201: basic electrical principles. Curr Surg. 2000;57(0149-7944 (Print)):261–4. PubMed PMID: 10930624.
7. Taheri A, Mansoori P, Sandoval LF, Feldman SR, Pearce D, Williford PM. Electrosurgery: part II. Technology, applications, and safety of electrosurgical devices. J Am Acad Dermatol. 2014;70(4):607.e1–12; quiz 619–20. https://doi.org/10.1016/j.jaad.2013.09.055. PubMed PMID: 24629362.
8. Fante RG, Fante RL. Perspective: the physical basis of surgical electrodissection. Ophthalmic Plast Reconstr Surg. 2003;19(0740-9303 (Print)):145–8. https://doi.org/10.1097/01.IOP.0000055825.19773.0E. PubMed PMID: 12644762.
9. Sebben JE. Electrosurgery principles: cutting current and cutaneous surgery—part I. J Dermatol Surg Oncol. 1988;14(0148-0812 (Print)):29–31. PubMed PMID: 3275701.
10. Palanker D, Vankov A, Jayaraman P. On mechanisms of interaction in electrosurgery. New J Phys [Internet]. 2008;10. Available from: ISI:000264869500008.
11. Noble WH, McClatchey KD, Douglass GD. A histologic comparison of effects of electrosurgical resection using different electrodes. J Prosthet Dent. 1976;35(5):575–9. PubMed PMID: 1063874.
12. Boughton RS, Spencer SK. Electrosurgical fundamentals. J Am Acad Dermatol. 1987;16(0190-9622 (Print)):862–7. PubMed PMID: 3571547.
13. Buzina DS, Lipozencic J. Electrosurgery—have we forgotten it? Acta Dermatovenerol Croat. 2007;15(1330-027X (Print)):96–102. PubMed PMID: 17631790.
14. Laughlin SA, Dudley DK. Electrosurgery. Clin Dermatol. 1992;10(0738-081X (Print)):285–90. PubMed PMID: 1483247.
15. Duffy S, Cobb GV. Practical electrosurgery. 1st ed. London: Chapman & Hall; 1995.
16. Eggleston JL, von Maltzahn WW. Electrosurgical devices. In: Bronzino JD, editor. The biomedical engineering handbook. Boca Raton: CRC Press; 2000.
17. Kalkwarf KL, Krejci RF, Edison AR. A method to measure operating variables in electrosurgery. J Prosthet Dent. 1979;42(5):566–70. PubMed PMID: 290807.
18. Strock MS. The rationale for electrosurgery. Oral Surg Oral Med Oral Pathol. 1952;5(11):1166–72. PubMed PMID: 13003151.
19. Elliott JA. Electrosurgery. Its use in dermatology, with a review of its development and technologic aspects. Arch Dermatol. 1966;94(0003-987X (Print)):340–50. PubMed PMID: 4952822.
20. Chino A, Karasawa T, Uragami N, Endo Y, Takahashi H, Fujita R. A comparison of depth of tissue injury caused by different modes of electrosurgical current in a pig colon model. Gastrointest Endosc. 2004;59(0016-5107 (Print)):374–9. PubMed PMID: 14997134.

21. Duffy S. The tissue and thermal effects of electrosurgery in the uterine cavity. Baillieres Clin Obstet Gynaecol. 1995;9(0950-3552 (Print)):261–77. PubMed PMID: 7554612.
22. Ruidiaz ME, Cortes-Mateos MJ, Sandoval S, Martin DT, Wang-Rodriguez J, Hasteh F, et al. Quantitative comparison of surgical margin histology following excision with traditional electrosurgery and a low-thermal-injury dissection device. J Surg Oncol. 2011;104(1096-9098 (Electronic)):746–54. https://doi.org/10.1002/jso.22012. PubMed PMID: 21744349.
23. Schoinohoriti OK, Chrysomali E, Iatrou I, Perrea D. Evaluation of lateral thermal damage and reepithelialization of incisional wounds created by CO(2)-laser, monopolar electrosurgery, and radiosurgery: a pilot study on porcine oral mucosa. Oral Surg Oral Med Oral Pathol Oral Radiol Endod. 2011;(1528-395X (Electronic)). https://doi.org/10.1016/j.tripleo.2011.06.016. PubMed PMID: 21906972.
24. Sebben JE. Electrosurgery principles: cutting current and cutaneous surgery—part II. J Dermatol Surg Oncol. 1988;14(0148-0812 (Print)):147–50. PubMed PMID: 3343421.
25. Aird LNF, Brown CJ. Systematic review and meta-analysis of electrocautery versus scalpel for surgical skin incisions. Am J Surg. 2012;204(2):216–21. https://doi.org/10.1016/j.amjsurg.2011.09.032. PubMed PMID: 22537473.
26. Bussiere RL. Principles of electrosurgery. Edmonds: Tektran Inc.; 1997.
27. Covidien [Internet]. Principles of electrosurgery. 2008 [cited 2013 Feb 2]. Available from: http://www.asit.org/assets/documents/Prinicpals_in_electrosurgery.pdf.

Chapter 5
Clinical Applications of Electrosurgery

Abstract Electrosurgery can provide electrocoagulation or electrosection in a variety of different surgical procedures. In dermatologic surgery, this flexible method can be used for selective destruction of the epidermis while preserving the reticular dermis, deep destruction of the epidermis and dermis, selective destruction of subcutaneous targets, bloodless cutting, hemostasis, or even for skin rejuvenation. Newer technologies and advances in this field provide more capabilities to this method, helping surgeons practice safer and more efficiently.

In this chapter, the term *mode* refers to the generator's output setting selected via the device interface. This selection determines the waveform of the current. The term *method* refers to the actual procedure performed. For example, a coagulation mode delivers an interrupted current, which can be used for performing any method, such as fulguration, contact coagulation, or cutting.

5.1 Review of Electrosurgical Modalities

5.1.1 Electrocoagulation

Key Points

- Coagulation can be performed in contact mode or spray (fulguration) mode. However, the term electrocoagulation is usually used to refer to electrocoagulation in contact mode.
- At the end of contact electrocoagulation, the more superficial coagulated tissues may dry out (desiccation). At this time, the current decreases or stops flowing; a popping sound may be heard; and sparking may occur through the dried, nonconductive layer, leading to the explosion and fragmentation of this layer.
- In the contact method, a fine-tip electrode can provide superficial electrocoagulation, while a large-tip electrode with a large contact area provides deep coagulation.
- A relatively slow coagulation using a relatively low power may provide a deeper burn than a short pulse of coagulation using a higher power.

A. Taheri et al., *Advanced Electrosurgery*,
https://doi.org/10.1007/978-3-032-28342-9_5

- Fulguration can provide a superficial coagulation if a relatively low power is used. It can cause deeper tissue damage if a relatively higher power is used or if the activated electrode is kept in a confined area for a longer period.

Electrocoagulation can be performed using different methods. Classical electrofulguration provides superficial coagulation. Contact coagulation can provide superficial or deep coagulation. A true desiccation can provide the deepest coagulation as deep as 5 mm or even more if larger-tip electrodes are used.

Electrofulguration is an easy procedure to perform and needs less training and mastery compared with contact coagulation. Performing contact coagulation needs a good understanding of the basics of electricity and electrosurgery. The advantages of contact coagulation over fulguration are its flexibility for providing a deeper coagulation, better hemostasis, less smoke, and theoretically less risk of infection spread through evaporated tissue particles [1]. One limitation of contact coagulation is that the depth of tissue destruction is not visible during the procedure. If the surgeon prefers not to coagulate the whole dermis, multiple passes of fulguration and curettage may give the surgeon better control over the depth of destruction.

The most common methods of application of the current for performing electrocoagulation are:

Method 1: Fulguration using the tip of a needle or knife-shaped electrode

In this method, the generator is activated, and then the tip of the electrode is brought near the tissue. Upon contact, sparks form (Fig. 5.1). The electrode is moved along the tissue surface at a speed sufficient to cause coagulation or hemostasis. The depth of injury depends on the output power of the generator and on the speed at which the electrode is moved along the surface. The slower the electrode moves on the tissue surface, the deeper the tissue injury. This method is mainly used for superficial coagulation or hemostasis of small surface areas.

Fulguration or coagulation modes of electrosurgical generators (interrupted waveforms) may provide larger sparks for covering a larger surface area than cutting mode with a continuous waveform can. Larger sparks can act like a larger brush or spray to speed up the procedure.

Method 2: Fulguration using the edge of a knife or blade electrode

This method is performed similarly to method 1. However, the large electrode acts like a large brush that can spray the sparks over a larger area with each pass of the electrode (Fig. 5.2). This method is used for superficial coagulation of large surface areas.

Any current waveform (fulguration, coagulation, cutting mode) can be used for this procedure. Using a high-power output, especially in cutting mode, may cause a cut if a part of the electrode comes in firm contact with tissue. This risk makes method 2 inferior to method 3, which is safer and easier to perform.

Method 3: Fulguration using a large-tip electrode, such as the flat side of a knife or blade electrode

In this method, the generator is activated, and then the flat side of a knife or blade electrode touches the target. Upon contact, sparks form (Fig. 5.3). The surgeon

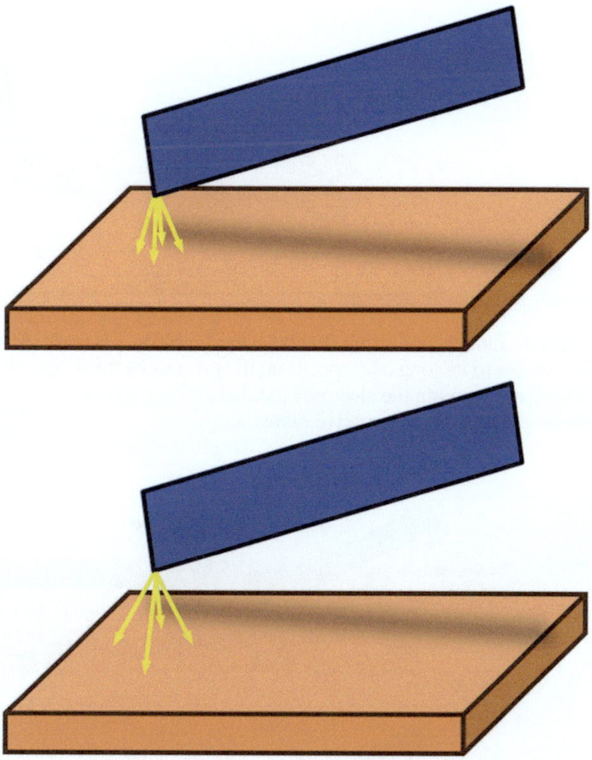

Fig. 5.1 Fulguration using the tip of a knife-shaped electrode. If a low-voltage current is used, the electrode needs to be near the tissue (top). A higher-pick voltage (e.g., fulguration mode) can provide larger sparks to enable the electrode to operate even if it is kept farther from the tissue. This setting can spray the current on a larger surface area (bottom)

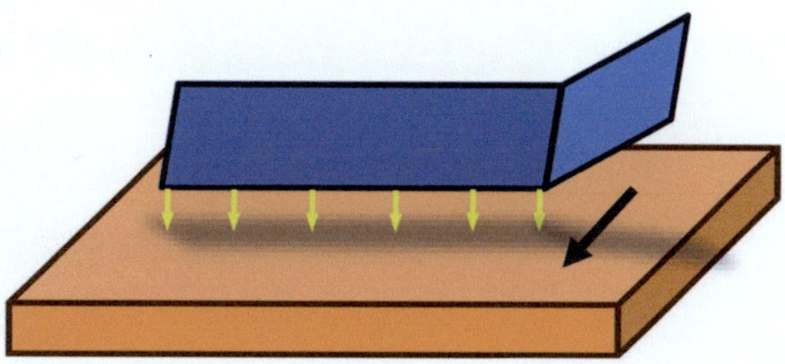

Fig. 5.2 Fulguration using the edge of a blade electrode. If the blade moves in a direction perpendicular to its long axis (black arrow), it can act like a large brush

applies enough pressure to keep all the electrode surfaces in good "contact" with the tissue. However, there is no direct physical contact between the electrode and the tissue. The gas produced from tissue explosions at the end of sparks keeps a gap and prevents the electrode from coming in direct contact with the tissue.

If the tissue surface is not flat, the surgeon may need to press the electrode firmer against the tissue for a better and more homogenous "contact." When a part of the electrode comes in direct contact with tissue, a higher current will be concentrated on that spot, causing more tissue explosion. This explosion pushes the electrode

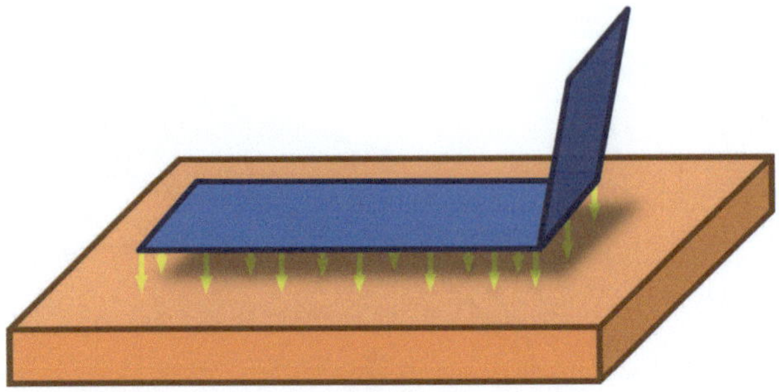

Fig. 5.3 Fulguration using the flat side of a blade electrode. Moving the blade in a direction perpendicular to its long axis speeds up the process by covering a larger area per unit of time. On the other hand, moving the electrode parallel and along its long axis can provide a deeper coagulation, because each spot will receive more energy

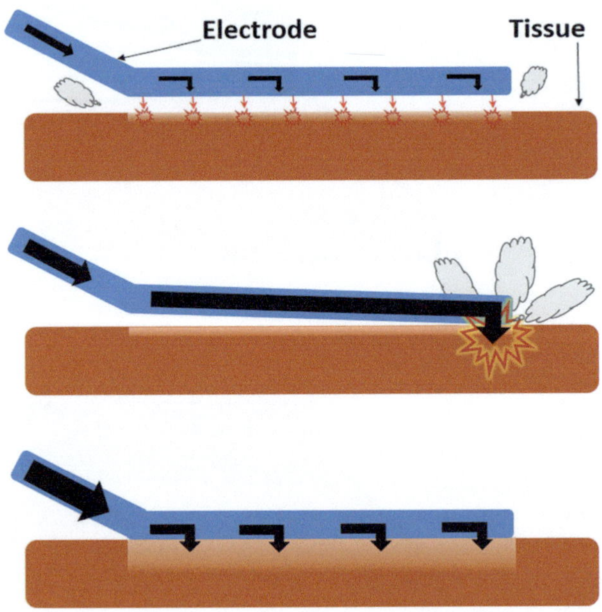

Fig. 5.4 Top: A large-tip electrode is used in fulguration mode. The surgeon applies enough pressure to keep the electrode in good "contact" with the tissue. However, the gas produced from sparks and tissue explosions keeps a gap and prevents the electrode from coming in direct contact with the tissue. Middle: If a part of the electrode touches the tissue, the circuit resistance falls, and a higher current will be concentrated on that spot, causing tissue explosion. This explosion pushes the electrode away from the tissue again, restarting fulguration. Bottom: If a large part of the electrode comes in contact with the tissue, no explosion may occur. With no explosion or spark, coagulation will continue in contact mode, and a higher current passes and causes a deep coagulation

away from the tissue again, restarting fulguration (Fig. 5.4). However, if the surgeon applies too much pressure and a large part of the electrode comes in contact with the tissue, or if the power output is relatively low, no explosion may occur. With no explosion or spark, coagulation will continue in contact mode and may cause deeper tissue damage than fulguration (Fig. 5.4). If it happens, the surgeon can pull the electrode off the tissue and restart the process.

When fulgurating using a large-tip electrode, the electrode is moved by the surgeon along the tissue surface at a speed sufficient to cause coagulation or hemostasis. This method can provide minimally deeper coagulation than previously mentioned methods 1 and 2 if all other parameters are the same. The depth of coagulation is still much less than contact coagulation using a large-tip electrode (Fig. 5.5).

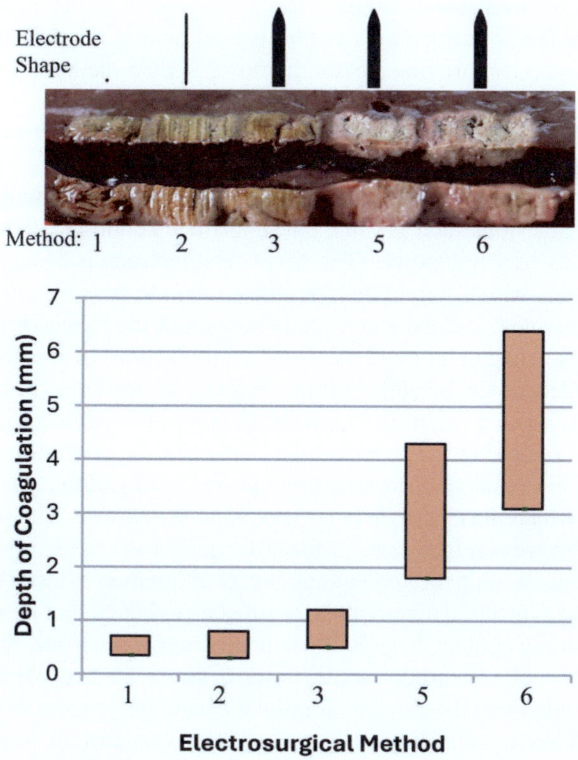

Fig. 5.5 Effects of electrocoagulation on bovine liver. (Source: Int J Dermatol. 2019 Dec;58(12):1472–6. With permission) [2]. Fulguration using the tip (method 1) or edge (method 2) of a knife-shaped electrode provides superficial coagulation (light-brown color change). Fulguration using the flat side of a knife-shaped electrode (method 3) provides marginally deeper coagulation. Coagulation in the contact method (method 5) is significantly deeper than fulguration. The depth of coagulation in this method is not homogeneous and is deepest near the tip of the electrode. Desiccation (method 6) provides the deepest coagulation

Coagulation using a fine-tip electrode (method 4) was not evaluated in this study

“Electrode shape” refers to the shape of the electrode–tissue contact area

In methods 2–6, the electrode was put on the tissue and moved on the tissue in a direction perpendicular to its long axis

Any current waveform (fulguration, coagulation, cutting mode) can be used for this procedure. To avoid the electrode sticking to tissue, this method needs a relatively high-power current to be dialed on the generator. Since there is a very high resistance to electricity in the gap between the tissue and the electrode, the actual current that passes the target tissue is low power even when high power is dialed on the unit. This is one of the reasons fulguration is known to be potentially more superficial than contact coagulation at the same dialed power setting.

A large-tip electrode is not likely to cut the tissue even when using a very high-power current. Therefore, the surgeon can safely push the electrode against the tissue for better and more homogeneous contact. This is an advantage of this method over method 2 when using a high power for fast coagulation of a large surface area. Inexperienced surgeons might be hesitant to use this method and may prefer method 1, which needs a lower-power output. The downside of using method 1 for the coagulation of a larger surface area is that it is slow and not as homogeneous as method 3. Method 3 can provide a better hemostasis than methods 1 and 2.

Method 4: Contact coagulation using a fine-tip electrode, such as the tip of a needle or knife-shaped electrode

This method is generally used for superficial coagulation of small epidermal or superficial dermal lesions such as small flat seborrheic keratoses. In this method, the generator is set to very low power. The tip of the electrode is brought into contact with the epidermis, which should be hydrated enough to pass the current. The generator is then activated, and the electrode is moved on the tissue surface at a speed sufficient to cause coagulation and softening (liquefaction) of the epidermis. Then the softened epidermis can be wiped off to see if the desired depth of destruction has been achieved. If using a sharp-tip electrode, the tip of the electrode can be used for scraping off and removing the coagulated tissue when the generator is off.

The depth of injury depends on the output power setting of the generator and also on the speed at which the electrode is moved along the surface. The slower the activated electrode moves on the tissue surface, the deeper the tissue injury.

If the epidermis is not hydrated enough, or if coagulation extends to desiccation, the epidermis may turn into a hard and dry substance that cannot be wiped off.

When performing contact coagulation using a fine-tip electrode, the direct physical contact between the electrode and the tissue is interrupted very frequently. When the active electrode loses its contact with moist tissue, the process will change from contact coagulation to fulguration. Using a continuous current (cutting mode) is preferred over an interrupted current (coagulation or fulguration mode) for this method because it does not cause large sparks when fulguration happens. However, some electrosurgical units may not have a very low dial setting for output power in their cutting mode.

This method may not work in the presence of blood. And even if it works, it is too slow to be used for hemostasis on a large oozing surface.

Method 5: Contact coagulation using an electrode with a large tissue interface, such as a disk- or ball-shaped electrode, or the flat side of a knife or blade electrode

The large surface of the electrode is brought into complete contact with hydrated tissue. The generator is then activated, and the electrode is moved along the tissue surface at a speed sufficient to cause coagulation. Alternatively, the surgeon may perform spot treatment by holding the electrode on one spot until the desired coagulation is achieved and then moving the electrode to the next spot.

A major disadvantage of contact coagulation using a large-tip electrode is that the coagulation at the electrode–tissue interface does not start homogenously. Coagulation starts along the perimeter and extremities of the electrode and may go deep into those areas before all the tissue in contact with the electrode coagulates (Fig. 5.6) [3]. Therefore, this method is not a good option for achieving superficial coagulation. A ball-shaped electrode may provide more homogenous coagulation on the electrode–tissue interface than a disk-shaped or knife-shaped electrode. When using a knife-shaped electrode, coagulation starts at the tip of the electrode and goes deep before the tissue in contact with the more proximal part of the electrode coagulates (Fig. 5.6).

The depth of injury using this method is much deeper than the previously mentioned methods, is not easily visible during the procedure, and is also hard to predict (Fig. 5.5). Therefore, this method may not be used where the skin is very close to a major nerve, artery, bone, cartilage, or joint, especially if the surgeon is not experienced. Deep contact coagulation can be used for the treatment of benign or malignant skin lesions or for effective hemostasis where a scar is acceptable.

Other than the size of the electrode tip, the depth of coagulation depends on the amount of energy delivered, which is the result of power setting and activation time. A relatively high-power setting that enables the surgeon to move the electrode on the tissue quickly can provide relatively more superficial coagulation than when a lower-power setting is used for a very slow coagulation (Fig. 5.7). This is the same concept that applies to the pulse duration of lasers.

When there is significant bleeding from a wound bed, using a small-tip electrode or a low-power setting may not work. Using a large-tip electrode and using a higher power may be more effective for hemostasis on a severely bleeding scalp wound. A ball-shaped electrode can be a good choice for this procedure. If using a knife-shaped electrode, the electrode can move on the wound bed parallel to its long axis to provide a more homogenous coagulation and hemostasis (Fig. 5.6). Again, fulguration using a large-tip electrode is an alternative to this method, when the plan is hemostasis with a more superficial coagulation.

Method 6: Desiccation using an electrode with a large tissue interface, such as a disk- or ball-shaped electrode or the flat side of a knife or blade electrode

This method is performed similarly to method 5. However, the electrode is moved over the tissue at a speed slow enough to result in boiling of the water within the tissue and bubble formation. An audible popping sound or sparking signifies the final stage of desiccation and the start of fulguration. If it happens, the generator

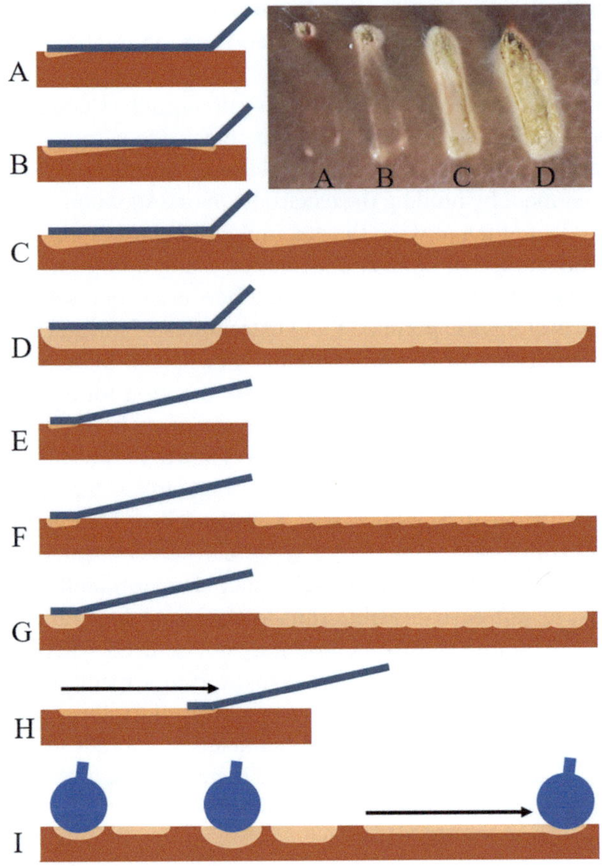

Fig. 5.6 Top: Spot contact coagulation using a long knife-shaped electrode in contact with tissue (**a**–**g**). Coagulation mainly starts from the tip of the electrode (**a**) and advances to involve the whole contact area (**b**, **c**). The coagulation will be more homogenous when desiccation happens (**d**). Middle: Using a shorter part of the electrode can provide more homogenous superficial coagulation (**e**, **f**) but may not have any advantage over a longer electrode if the plan is for a deep desiccation (**d**, **g**). Moving a knife-shaped electrode like a brush along its long axis on the tissue for a relatively superficial coagulation (**h**) can provide a more homogenous effect than when using the spot method (**f**). Bottom: Using a ball-shaped electrode can provide more homogeneous contact coagulation. Depending on the size of the ball, this method can be used for relatively superficial or deep coagulation in spot or brush methods (**i**)
Since desiccation can provide homogenous coagulation (**d**), a large desiccating electrode can move like a brush in any direction on tissue. However, many surgeons may find it easier to do spot treatment

should be deactivated, the tissue should be made moist again, and the sequence should be repeated. Alternatively, the surgeon can perform the procedure using the spot method (see below) rather than sliding the electrode on the surface. Desiccation is the deepest stage of coagulation, with a more homogenous and more predictable depth of injury on the contact area compared with method 5. This method is mainly used for cancer surgery after curettage to destroy a layer of the surrounding tissue.

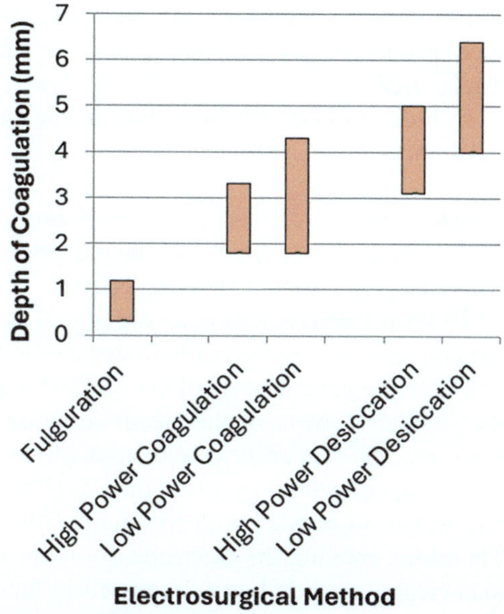

Fig. 5.7 An in vitro study on bovine liver comparing the depth of coagulation according to the electrosurgical method when using a large-tip electrode. Color change in tissue was considered as coagulation. (Unpublished author's study)

A relatively low-power setting and a long activation time (slow movement of the electrode on tissue) can provide a slow desiccation that is associated with the deepest coagulation. A higher power setting that reaches the point of tissue desiccation quickly and allows the surgeon to move faster along the tissue can provide less depth of injury compared with slow desiccation (Fig. 5.7) [4–7].

5.1.1.1 Contact Coagulation Using a Large-Tip Electrode: Spot Treatment Versus the Brush Method

Contact coagulation can be achieved using two methods: spot treatment or the brush method. Both methods can use a ball-shaped electrode. Alternatively, a knife-shaped electrode is bent, and the flat side of the electrode comes in contact with tissue.

Spot treatment (pulse) method: The electrode comes in good contact with the tissue and stays in place. Then the generator is activated to provide coagulation. After discontinuing the current, the electrode is removed and placed on an adjacent area on the target, and the procedure continues.

To keep the coagulation as superficial as possible, a relatively small ball-shaped electrode can be used. The output power of the generator should be at a minimum, just enough to provide coagulation or hemostasis with a very short pulse of energy (less than a second) at each spot. If a very short pulse cannot provide hemostasis before producing sparks, the duration of active contact (pulse duration) may need to be increased, while the power output is decreased. A longer pulse duration increases the depth of coagulation (Fig. 5.7).

For deeper coagulation, an electrode with a larger electrode–tissue interface, such as a larger ball-shaped electrode or the flat side of a knife-shaped electrode, can be used.

In order to keep the procedure faster and potentially more homogeneous, the brush method can be tried.

Brush method: A large-tip electrode comes into good contact with the tissue. Then the generator is activated, and the electrode moves like a brush on the wound bed while the generator is delivering energy.

To keep the coagulation as superficial as possible, similar to the spot treatment method, a relatively small ball-shaped electrode can be used. Again, the output power of the generator should be sufficient to yield coagulation or hemostasis with the swift movement of the electrode along the tissue. The larger the ball-shaped electrode, the deeper the coagulation will be. If using the flat side of a knife-shaped electrode, coagulation starts at the tip of the electrode and goes deep before the tissue that is in contact with the more proximal parts of the electrode coagulates. Therefore, moving the electrode on tissue in a direction perpendicular to its long axis cannot provide homogenous coagulation unless it is used up to the stage of desiccation (Fig. 5.6). If only a small part of the electrode at its tip is used in contact with tissue, it can provide a more homogenous and potentially more superficial coagulation compared with when a long part of the electrode comes in contact with tissue. Moving the knife-shaped electrode on the tissue surface parallel to its long axis can provide a more homogenous coagulation than moving it in a direction perpendicular to its long axis (Fig. 5.6).

If sparking (fulguration) happens during contact coagulation, it means that the electrode is not in good contact with the tissue. The generator should be deactivated. If the tissue is dry and desiccated, it can be moistened using saline or gauze soaked with blood. Then, the electrode comes into good contact with moist tissue again, and the generator is activated.

If the tissue boils and makes a popping sound, it means that a deep coagulation has happened. When desiccation happens, the procedure changes from contact coagulation to fulguration and continues in fulguration mode as long as sparking is observed. Continuing fulguration on a previously desiccated or coagulated tissue may cause explosion and disruption of the coagulated tissue, which may interfere with good hemostasis. On the other hand, continuing fulguration on freshly desiccated hot tissue may cause deeper injury [4–6].

One potential complication of deep electrocoagulation is damage to subcutaneous structures such as nerves, vessels, or cartilage. Because subcutaneous structures and the extent of coagulation or desiccation are not visible during procedures, this complication may not be detected during surgery. To minimize the risk of damage to underlying structures, saline or lidocaine can be injected into the superficial subcutaneous plane underneath the target skin to elevate and separate it from the deeper structures.

Electrocoagulation of Pedunculated Skin Lesions or Bleeding Arteries Using Forceps

This procedure can be performed using bipolar forceps or using surgical forceps or a surgical clamp connected to an active electrode in monopolar mode. The difference in the final results is that, in bipolar mode, the tissue between the tips of the forceps is coagulated, while, in monopolar mode, the tissue between the forceps and the patient's body is coagulated without affecting the tissue that is held between the tips. The bipolar method can be more accurate in focusing coagulation on the target; however, it may not be available during a fast-paced surgical procedure.

To perform bipolar coagulation, the target is held between the tips of a bipolar forceps, and then the generator is activated. The current passes until the boiling of water is heard. A popping sound indicates desiccation. Further passage of current may cause fulguration and fragmentation of the coagulated tissue that may interfere with the hemostasis of a bleeding artery. A relatively low-power continuous current (cutting mode) is the preferred current in order to avoid large sparks.

If the bipolar forceps are activated before touching the target tissue, it causes fulguration, which leads to superficial coagulation on the surface of the target, rather than coagulation of the whole tissue held between the tips.

To perform monopolar coagulation using surgical forceps, the target is held between the tips of the forceps. The active electrode touches the forceps, and the current passes until the boiling of water or a popping sound is heard.

5.1.2 Electrosection

Key Points

- A thin needle-shaped electrode and a continuous cutting current (cut mode) can provide a pure cut with relatively clean incision walls and little hemostasis. Pure cutting of the tissue should be brisk with the lowest possible power setting.
- Blend cutting can be performed using an interrupted current (blend or coagulation mode). A thick electrode or a slow cut can also increase the coagulation depth on the incision walls and improve hemostasis.

Electrosection is used when the surgeon needs to achieve hemostasis immediately after the incision. This procedure is commonly used for endoscopic surgeries where hemostasis cannot be achieved using pressure or other methods. In dermatologic surgeries, electrosection can save time when cutting tissues with high blood supply, such as the scalp or eyelids.

To perform a pure cut, a needle-shaped electrode is used in pure cut mode. The generator is activated, and the electrode touches the target. The cutting of the tissue should be brisk with the lowest possible power setting that enables the active electrode to cut fast. If the electrode sticks to the tissue and does not cut fast, the power output needs to be increased. If there is too much sparking, the power needs to be decreased.

Using a thicker electrode, using an interrupted current, or cutting slowly provides a blend cut with more coagulation on the incision walls, better hemostasis, and potentially more scarring.

5.2 Electrosurgery Versus Other Surgical Methods

5.2.1 Electrosection Versus Scalpel Surgery

Electrosection provides a means of cutting tissue in place of a scalpel. The major advantage of electrosection is that hemostasis is achieved immediately upon incision by coagulation on either side of the incision wall. Therefore, electrosection can significantly reduce surgical time and blood loss from skin incisions [8].

A loop-shaped electrosection electrode can be used for shaving dome-shaped benign lesions on the scalp, where bleeding can be an issue, and dressing is not easy. To provide more effective and longer-lasting hemostasis, an interrupted current can be used for a blend cut.

There is conflicting evidence in studies comparing electrosection versus scalpel with respect to surgical outcomes such as postoperative pain, infection, wound healing, and scar formation. While many studies support better outcomes using scalpel surgery, there is also literature favoring electrosection [9–12]. Although the general concept is to avoid electrosection for cutting skin when primary closure is planned, review articles and meta-analyses have shown no significant difference in wound infection rates or scar cosmesis between surgical wounds created with electrosection versus traditional scalpel surgery [8]. A pure cut may have outcomes closer to scalpel surgery compared with a blend cut.

Collateral tissue damage associated with electrosection results in histologic distortion of surgical margins, including carbonization at the excision margin, vessel thrombosis, and collagen denaturation [13, 14]. Cellular changes may include vacuolar degeneration, shrunken and shriveled cell outlines with condensation and elongation of the nuclei, or fusion of cells into a structureless homogeneous mass with a hyalinized appearance [15]. In frozen sections, normal structures may mimic tumors such as basal cell carcinoma [16]. For specimens requiring histopathological analysis, especially during the excision of tumors that require the margins to be assessed, scalpel surgery is preferred. Using pure cut mode for electrosection may result in less thermal tissue damage than using blend mode.

5.2.2 Electrosection Versus CO2 Laser Surgery

Like electrosection, the CO2 laser can provide coagulation of the incision walls and hemostasis. Both techniques, especially electrosection, are operator-dependent and cannot be standardized. Therefore, it is not easy to compare these methods in clinical settings. There is conflicting evidence in studies comparing the depth of collateral injury and final surgical results using these modalities. While some studies show more collateral coagulation using CO2 lasers, others report the opposite results [11, 12, 17–22]. Compared to a CO2 laser, electrosurgery is generally less expensive, does not require eye protection, and is more available.

5.2.3 Electrocoagulation Versus Excision

Electrocoagulation and destruction of benign or malignant skin tumors is an alternative to excision when primary closure is not planned. Instead of removing the unwanted tissue, the surgeon burns the tissue and leaves it in place for hemostasis. The process is significantly faster than excision and primary closure or excision and hemostasis of the base. The main limitation of this method is that the depth of the coagulated tissue cannot be seen during the surgery; therefore, in inexperienced hands, it may not be as predictable as surgical excision, where the surgeon can plan and see the extent and depth of tissue removal.

In order to have a better estimate and visibility of the depth of coagulation, a superficial coagulation can be performed. Then the coagulated layer is removed using curette. Then, the procedure is repeated until the desired depth of tissue destruction is achieved.

5.2.4 Electrocoagulation Versus Cryosurgery

For treating benign or premalignant epidermal lesions such as seborrheic keratoses and actinic keratosis, cryosurgery has the advantage of being faster to perform, less painful for the patient, with no need for anesthesia, and having less risk of scar formation, compared with electrosurgery.

Cryosurgery is also preferred for the treatment of viral warts, where electrosurgery can potentially cause the spread of the virus through surgical smoke.

Electrosurgery, especially if combined with curettage, is more reliable than cryotherapy for treating thicker and deeper skin lesions and for epidermal cancers such as basal cell carcinoma or squamous cell carcinoma [23]. A clinical trial comparing cryotherapy versus electrocoagulation after curettage of minimally invasive basal and squamous cell carcinomas showed no statistically significant difference in cure rate or scar formation [24]. However, hemostasis was probably easier to achieve with electrocoagulation.

When treating a very small epidermal lesion on dark skin, electrosurgery has the advantage of being able to focus the destruction on a small target. Cryosurgery is harder to focus or concentrate on a small area and usually causes more inflammation and dyspigmentation on the skin around the target compared with electrosurgery. Therefore, electrosurgery may be preferred over cryosurgery on a dark skin.

5.2.5 Electrocoagulation for Achieving Hemostasis

Electrocoagulation is a fast method of achieving hemostasis. It can be used to seal bleeding vessels or for oozing surfaces.

Hemostasis of a bleeding vessel can be performed using a bipolar electrode or by clamping the vessel and passing a monopolar current through the surgical clamp or forceps. The current should be passed until the tissue is completely coagulated. The tissue changes color, a popping sound may be heard, or a spark may be seen at the end of coagulation when desiccation happens; at this time, the current flow should be stopped. Care should be taken to prevent spark formation that can cause tissue fragmentation at the end of coagulation. A relatively low-power continuous current (cutting mode) is the preferred current in order to prevent large spark formation. Some modern electrosurgical devices used for endoscopic procedures have bipolar modes equipped with an automated system that discontinues the current at the time of desiccation and just before any spark formation. These devices sense the electrical resistance of tissue between the tips of the bipolar forceps and drop off the current when this resistance increases at the time of desiccation and tissue drying. Bipolar or monopolar forceps should not be activated before coming in contact with the bleeding tissue. Touching the tissue with activated forceps causes fulguration, which provides superficial damage to the outer layer of the vessel, rather than coagulating the whole tissue between the forceps tips.

For hemostasis of an oozing surface, contact coagulation or fulguration may be used. Fulguration provides a thin layer of coagulated tissue unless the surgeon keeps the activated electrode over a specific location for a long time, which leads to heat conduction in the tissue and deep coagulation. A typical superficial fulguration may control minimal capillary oozing with minimal depth of damage to the tissue. However, this thin, fulgurated layer is not stable and may bleed with minimal trauma. Aggressive wiping of the fulgurated area should be avoided if possible because it can cause disruption of the coagulated layer. For fulguration of a large surface area, using a large-tip electrode, such as the flat side of a knife-shaped electrode, improves the efficiency of the procedure compared with a fine-tip electrode.

Contact coagulation can also be performed using an electrode with a large contact surface area, such as a ball-shaped electrode or the flat side of a knife-shaped electrode. This method of contact coagulation usually results in a significantly deeper coagulation and better hemostasis than fulguration; however, it may adversely affect postoperative and aesthetic outcomes.

To optimize hemostasis, the blood should be suctioned or wiped off the operative field, as blood diffuses the current away from the target tissue and interferes with coagulation. If oozing cannot be controlled with pressure, contact coagulation using a large-tip electrode may work better than fulguration. A bloodless operative field is also essential for cutting and coagulation. Using a very high-power output can provide a deep coagulation or even cutting in a bloody field; however, the boiling blood around the electrode–tissue contact area may cause coagulation of a larger surface than the target. Electrocautery may function in bloody environments, although not as effectively as in dry fields.

5.3 Electrosurgery for Hair Removal

- Hair removal can be performed using a needle electrode that enters the hair follicle and delivers an electrical current. The needle can apply a direct (galvanic) electrical current (electrolysis) or an alternating electrosurgical current (thermolysis).
- In electrolysis, the resulting electrochemical reaction around the electrode destroys the hair follicle. The process is very slow and time-consuming.
- In thermolysis, an electrosurgical alternating current destroys the follicle by thermal damage (electrocoagulation). This process is much faster than electrolysis; however, there is more risk of damage to the dermis around the hair follicle and scar formation.

The first report on using electricity for hair removal was published in 1875. The author described the use of a direct (galvanic) current to electrochemically destroy the germinative cells of the hair follicle. In this method, a needle-shaped electrode is inserted in the hair follicle, and a low-power direct current is passed through the needle for a few seconds to minutes. In the hair follicle, at the electrode–tissue interface, a chemical reaction called electrolysis occurs and causes the destruction of a thin layer of tissue around the electrode [25–28]. The chemically damaged tissue around the needle may not show any color or consistency change at the time of the procedure; however, it undergoes necrosis in a few hours to days.

In electrolysis, the needle is attached to the negative electrode. Iron tattooing on the treatment area has been reported after attaching steel needles to the positive electrode.

Electrolysis is a slow process and may require 30 seconds to well over 1 min to produce the desired effect on each hair. In order to increase the rate at which hairs could be destroyed, a multiple-needle technique was developed. This method involves the sequential placing and removal of multiple electrodes while always maintaining several active electrodes within the patient. The multiple-needle method was very complicated and was never widely used.

In an attempt to make the hair removal process faster, high-frequency electrosurgical currents were used to cause thermal damage to the hair follicle. In this method, which is called thermolysis, a needle-shaped electrode is inserted in the hair follicle, and a low-power electrosurgical current is passed through the needle. Thermolysis, which is the same as electrocoagulation, is faster and more practical to perform than electrolysis. However, it is more painful, less effective, and more likely to cause scarring than electrolysis. Because of being more practical, thermolysis became the most popular method of permanent hair removal in the 1940s and was used extensively until the 1990s, when lasers dominated the market and practically put an end to the use of electrical currents for permanent hair removal.

There are two methods of performing thermolysis. In the *slow* technique, a low-power current is passed over for a few seconds. In the *flash* technique, a relatively higher power is delivered via a preset timer on the machine at a duration of less than 1 second. Several pulses may be necessary to achieve hair follicle destruction. The safety and efficacy of the two delivery methods have not been compared in any clinical trial.

Between 1940 and 1990, some devices were developed that used a "blend" of a direct current and an alternating current to provide a combination of electrolysis and thermolysis. There are no clinical trials comparing these devices with devices that use only one current type.

Practical Pearls for Performing Electrolysis or Thermolysis

The hairs in the treatment area are shaved 3–10 days before the procedure. The hairs that grow after shaving are in the growth phase (anagen phase). These hairs have their shafts in the hair follicle down to the hair papilla. Therefore, by inserting an electrode into the follicle parallel to the hair shaft, we can reach the whole length of the follicle and all the germinal cells in it [28].

In both electrolysis and thermolysis, a needle-shaped electrode with a round tip is used. The needle tip is rounded to decrease the likelihood of puncturing the hair follicle. The needle is inserted in the hair follicle, paralleling the hair shaft. Excessive force should not be applied to avoid puncturing the hair follicle. When a gentle resistance is felt, probably the hair bulb has been reached, and the current is turned on with a foot pedal.

In thermolysis, gentle traction is applied to the hair with a fine tweezer during the application of the current or after discontinuing the current. When root destruction is complete, the hair can be pulled out with minimal traction. If the hair does not come out easily, it means that the needle has not been inserted down to the hair bulb, the needle has been out of the hair follicle, or not enough electrical energy was used. Repeating the process on the same follicle is not recommended. The operator should try new follicles to find the optimal electrical energy and activation time. After finding the optimal energy for the destruction of a few hair follicles, the same amount of energy can be used for the rest of the hairs in the treatment area without any need to pull them out of the skin.

Some patients with curly hair may have curved hair follicles that are not easy to enter using a needle-shaped electrode. Electrolysis or thermolysis does not have good results in these patients.

Minimal edema or redness around the hair follicles is normal during or after the procedure. Significant swelling, burning, or sparking are the signs of overtreatment and are considered risk factors for developing scars. Overtreatment can cause severe disfiguring scars in the treatment area and should be avoided.

If the hair density in the treatment area is high, the chance of scar formation will increase. In these patients, treating all hair in one session should be avoided. At least a 2-mm distance between the treated hair follicles is recommended. The remaining hairs can be treated in the next sessions if no scar formation is observed.

The treatment sessions should be at least 1 month apart. The redness and inflammation from the previous session should be completely resolved before the next session, and no scar should be observed.

Efforts have been made to develop needles that would concentrate electrical currents to the mid- and deep follicles, avoiding the epidermis. A thin needle with a bulbous tip can theoretically burn the deeper parts of the follicle better. Proximally insulated needles may also protect the epidermis and superficial parts of the follicle while destroying most of the deeper parts. Because the length of the hair follicles is not the same, the proximally insulated needles may work for some follicles, may not protect the epidermis in the shorter follicles, and may prevent destruction of the mid-follicle in longer follicles. There is no clinical trial comparing insulated needles with non-insulated ones.

Several devices have been marketed for self-electroepilation. Those employing tweezers as active electrodes for delivering the current are no more effective than plucking the hairs.

5.4 Electrosurgery in the Treatment of Malignant Skin Tumors

Curettage and Electrocoagulation

Curettage and electrocoagulation is a relatively easy-to-perform, fast, low-risk, and inexpensive treatment method for less aggressive malignant skin tumors. This method can be used to treat multiple lesions in a single session in a shorter time and with relatively less stress to the patient compared with excision and primary closure or graft.

Most skin cancers are not encapsulated and infiltrate into normal surrounding tissues. Extensions of tumoral invasion into the normal tissue almost always go beyond the clinically visible borders of the lesion. This is the reason surgeons excise the cancers with a margin of the normal-looking surrounding tissues. With more infiltrative tumors, a wider margin of surrounding tissue should be removed to achieve an acceptable cure rate. This process sacrifices some of the normal tissue and makes a wound larger than the actual tumor. A great advantage of curettage over surgical excision arises from the ability of a semi-sharp curette to differentiate and remove a friable tumor from the normal surrounding tissue with minimal sacrifice of normal skin [29]. A semi-sharp curette may not be able to remove all small extensions of the tumor in the surrounding tissue; therefore, another destructive measure is usually used to remove or destroy a layer of surrounding tissue after removing the tumor mass. Some surgeons may use a sharp curette to perform another curettage and remove a layer of surrounding tissue. Some surgeons may use chemical cautery or hot iron electrocautery to provide hemostasis and destruction of the curetted wound bed. Electrosurgery has the advantage of providing effective hemostasis as well as flexibility to provide different depths of destruction on the wound bed after curettage. A relatively thin destruction can be achieved using fulguration, while desiccation can provide deep coagulation.

Most subtypes of basal cell carcinomas and superficial nonaggressive forms of squamous cell carcinomas have been treated using curettage and electrocoagulation with very promising cure rates. These tumors tend to have somewhat more friable tissue than the surrounding stroma.

The main disadvantage of curettage and electrocoagulation is that the remaining open wound may take more time to heal compared with an excision and primary closure. This wound may leave a scar, which can be cosmetically unacceptable to some patients.

The other disadvantage of curettage and electrocoagulation is that this method is more operator-dependent than surgical excision. An inexperienced surgeon may not perform an effective curettage to remove all the tumoral tissue or may fail to provide an ideal depth of coagulation.

5.4.1 Basal Cell Carcinoma

Basal cell carcinoma (BCC) may be the most common malignant tumor treated with curettage and electrocoagulation in dermatology practice. Multiple small BCCs can be treated using this fast method in a single surgical session.

To our knowledge, no randomized trials comparing curettage and electrocoagulation with other surgical treatments for BCC have been published. However, based on the limited available data from case series, curettage and electrocoagulation is considered as effective as surgical excision for small, low-risk tumors (Table 5.1) [30].

Recurrence rates for BCC after curettage and electrocoagulation range from 1% to 27% in different studies. Although the recurrence rate is influenced by anatomical location, histopathological growth pattern, and size of the tumor [31–38], the main reason for the difference in recurrence rate in previously reported studies may be the difference in surgical method. Studies that reported the highest cure rates destroyed a wider peripheral margin around the initial curettage [35, 39–42]. Repeating curettage and electrocoagulation (three passes versus one pass) also improved tumor removal [43].

Table 5.1 National Comprehensive Cancer Network stratification of low-risk versus high-risk basal cell carcinoma [30]

Risk factors associated with the recurrence of basal cell carcinoma (BCC). A BCC with none of the following risk factors is considered low risk	
Tumor characteristics	Any BCC in high-risk sites: central face, eyelids, eyebrows, periorbital skin, nose, lips, chin, mandible, preauricular and postauricular skin/sulci, temple, ear, genitalia, hands, and feet
	BCC >1-cm diameter in medium-risk sites: cheeks, forehead, scalp, neck, and pretibia
	BCC >2-cm diameter in low-risk sites: trunk and extremities (excluding hands, feet, nail units, pretibia, and ankles)
	Poorly defined tumor borders
	Locally recurrent BCC after primary therapy
	Immunosuppression
	Site of prior radiation therapy
Histology	High-risk histologic subtypes: morpheaform, sclerosing, infiltrative, basosquamous (metatypical), or micronodular features in any portion of the tumor (nodular, superficial, keratotic, infundibulocystic, and fibroepithelioma of Pinkus are considered low-risk pathologic subtypes)
	Perineural involvement

The recurrence rate is more predictable after surgical excision than after curettage and electrocoagulation. The recurrence rate of BCC after surgical excision ranges from 1% to 8% in previous studies, depending on the surgical margins [44–46]. Excision with a 3-mm peripheral surgical margin will clear the tumor in 85% of cases, while a 4–5-mm peripheral margin will increase the peripheral clearance rate to approximately 95% [47–49]. With excisions, surgical margins can be drawn and executed relatively accurately. In contrast, the depth of tissue coagulation and destruction of a tumor bed (which is equivalent to surgical margins) is not visible and cannot be planned or predicted easily with curettage and electrocoagulation unless the surgeon has a good understanding of electrosurgical methods. Depth of injury in electrocoagulation depends on many factors, including output power, size of the electrode tip, speed of movement of the electrode on the tissue or activation time, and the method of delivering the current (contact coagulation versus fulguration) [4].

5.4.2 Cutaneous Squamous Cell Carcinoma

Curettage and electrocoagulation is a commonly used method for the treatment of low-risk cutaneous squamous cell carcinoma (cSCC) (Table 5.2). However, no large randomized clinical trial has been performed to compare curettage and

Table 5.2 National Comprehensive Cancer Network stratification of low-risk versus high-risk cutaneous squamous cell carcinoma [50, 54, 56]

Risk factors associated with local recurrence and/or metastasis of cutaneous squamous cell carcinoma (cSCC). A cSCC with none of the following risk factors is considered low risk	
Tumor characteristics	Any cSCC in high-risk sites: central face, eyelids, eyebrows, periorbital skin, nose, lips, chin, mandible, preauricular and postauricular skin/sulci, temple, ear, genitalia, hands, and feet
	cSCC >1-cm diameter in medium-risk sites: cheeks, forehead, scalp, neck, and pretibia
	cSCC >2-cm diameter in low-risk sites: trunk and extremities (excluding hands, feet, nail units, pretibia, and ankles)
	Poorly defined borders
	cSCC exhibiting rapid growth
	Neurologic symptoms
	Locally recurrent cSCC after primary therapy
	Immunosuppression
	Site of prior radiation therapy, prior chronic wound, or prior chronic inflammatory process
Histology	Depth >4 mm
	Poorly differentiated
	High-risk histologic subtypes: adenoid (acantholytic), adenosquamous (showing mucin production), desmoplastic, spindle-cell, or metaplastic (carcinosarcomatous) subtypes
	Perineural or vascular invasion

electrocoagulation with other treatment modalities. Different recurrence rates have been reported in different studies for this procedure. The recurrence rate of cSCC after curettage and electrocoagulation has been estimated to be between 1.7% and 4% in review articles [50, 51]. A systematic review of eight retrospective series of variable follow-up periods revealed a recurrence rate of 1.7% (95% confidence interval: 0.5–3.4) [51]. Small, individual studies suggested higher recurrence rates for lesions greater than 2 cm in diameter or located on the ear. Recurrence in the lesions larger than 2 cm was 11.8% (95% confidence interval: 1.4–36.4%) compared with 0.4% (95% confidence interval: 0.0–2.1%) in the lesions smaller than 2 cm [51, 52]. One study separated results according to the number of treatment cycles used with no recurrences after more aggressive surgeries with either two or three cycles of curettage and electrocoagulation [53].

In experienced hands, curettage and electrocoagulation can have a cure rate near 100% for the treatment of low-risk cSCCs (Table 5.2) [53–55]. Although the presence of any single one of the mentioned risk factors may increase the recurrence rate of the tumor after any treatment method, there is no strong clinical evidence favoring surgical excision over curettage and electrocoagulation for high-risk cSCCs; therefore, none of the known risk factors is an absolute contraindication for performing curettage and electrocoagulation. Performing a very aggressive curettage and then a very deep electrodesiccation can increase the cure rate in any case. However, for a very high-risk cSCC, especially a poorly differentiated cSCC that has a higher metastasis rate, excision is the preferred method, because it can provide tissue for histopathological examination of the margins for confirmation of complete removal.

5.4.3 Squamous Cell Carcinoma In Situ or Bowen's Disease

Squamous cell carcinoma in situ or Bowen's disease is considered a low-risk tumor regardless of location or size [56, 57]. Considering the relatively lower risk of metastasis associated with Bowen's disease, less aggressive treatment options are more commonly used for this tumor compared with the more aggressive types of squamous cell carcinoma. Superficially destructive therapies have been used with limited published data available. A large retrospective study showed promising results for curettage and fulguration comparable to elliptical excision. In this study, cryotherapy was associated with the highest recurrence rate (5-year recurrence of 13.4%), followed by topical 5-fluorouracil (9%) and shave excision (9%). Curettage and fulguration (6.5%), Mohs micrographic surgery (6.3%), and elliptical excision (5.5%) had lower 5-year recurrence rates [58]. A clinical trial showed that curettage and electrocoagulation was superior to cryotherapy and had a recurrence rate of 9% [23]. Other studies using curettage and electrocoagulation gave a wide range of recurrence rates from 2% to 20% [59].

The relatively higher recurrence rate of squamous cell carcinoma in situ after curettage and electrocoagulation compared with invasive squamous cell carcinoma may be due to the behavior of the surgeons. The treating physician may perform any procedure less aggressively when treating a slow-growing, nonaggressive tumor compared with when treating a highly malignant cancer.

The British Association of Dermatologists has recommended curettage and electrocoagulation as one of the first-line treatments for squamous cell carcinoma in situ even on the face. This association does not recommend curettage and electrocoagulation for this indication on fingers or for large tumors on poor healing sites [59].

5.4.4 *Curettage and Electrocoagulation for BCC and cSCC in High-Risk Anatomic Areas*

Curettage and electrocoagulation for BCCs and cSCCs in high-risk anatomic areas have been associated with a higher recurrence rate in some studies [50, 60]. These high-risk anatomic areas include the head and neck, genitalia, hands, feet, and pretibial area. To our knowledge, there is no unique biological or tissue specification that makes the skin in these areas significantly different from the trunk or proximal extremities. And we are not aware of any genetic difference between BCCs and cSCCs in these high-risk areas and the ones on low-risk skin. It has been suggested that the discrepancy between recurrence rates in high-risk and low-risk areas may be due to a different tumor invasion pattern in these areas. However, the observation that a standard surgical excision of these tumors in the centrofacial area yields the same recurrence rate as elsewhere makes that explanation less likely. One interesting observation is that the list of high-risk anatomic areas includes all areas that have a sensitive underlying structure or are considered not acceptable for scar formation. Therefore, the main difference between the high-risk and low-risk areas may be in the eyes of the surgeons and the risk they accept.

The most likely reason for the discrepancy between the recurrence rate after curettage and electrocoagulation in high-risk and low-risk areas may be surgical technique. Concern about scarring or damage to the underlying structures may lead the surgeon to perform the procedures more gently and conservatively with less depth of destruction, which may lead to a greater chance of recurrence. The effect of the behavior and experience of surgeons on the cure rate after curettage and electrocoagulation have been shown in previous studies. In one study, resident physicians had recurrence rates of 10.8%, while a more experienced physician's rate was 2.6%, despite the fact that the experienced surgeon was treating larger and more difficult tumors [19]. Another study showed that a relatively aggressive curettage and electrocoagulation (repeating four or five cycles of curettage and electrocoagulation) performed by experts can have a cure rate of 99% (95% CI, 97–100%) for BCCs in high-risk areas of the face [35].

Some authors consider curettage and electrocoagulation less effective for BCC and cSCC on terminal-hair-bearing skin because of potential follicular extension of the tumor [30]. Although terminal-hair-bearing skin may not be a surgeon's favorite place to perform curettage and electrocoagulation, available published clinical data does not show any difference in recurrence rates after curettage and electrocoagulation between terminal-hair-bearing skin and the skin with no terminal hairs [50, 57]. Surgeons frequently find it harder to differentiate and remove friable tumoral tissues from normal surrounding tissues using a curette on these anatomic areas, because a semi-sharp curette does not cut the hair shafts and therefore does not work at all. A sharp curette that can cut hair shafts may cut the normal tissue as well and therefore may not be able to differentiate between the tumor and normal tissue.

An experienced surgeon knows that using a curette on skin with terminal hairs is not as easy as on sun-damaged friable skin with no terminal hair. The curette should be sharper and should be used in a more aggressive way to remove the tumoral tissue, the surrounding skin, and the hair shafts while avoiding overtreatment. Removal of the electrocoagulated tissue before repeating the procedure also needs a sharp curette in this setting.

5.4.5 Deep Basal Cell Carcinomas or Squamous Cell Carcinomas Reaching Subcutaneous Tissue

Some authors and surgeons believe that curettage and electrocoagulation is not a reliable or preferred treatment if the subcutaneous layer is reached during curettage. Those authors recommend the treatment be changed to excision in that setting. Although this is a good recommendation for first-year dermatology or surgery residents with limited surgical experience, an experienced surgeon who can differentiate normal from abnormal subcutaneous tissue might be able to remove a layer of subcutaneous fat the same way as during surgical excision and then perform a classical curettage and electrocoagulation on the edges of the dermis. The surgeon also should consider that wound healing may be slower when there is no dermis at the base of the wound to support epidermal growth and reepithelialization. To our knowledge, there is no clinical data or strong evidence against using curettage and electrocoagulation when the subcutaneous fat is reached.

5.4.6 Methods of Performing Curettage and Electrocoagulation for Basal Cell Carcinoma and Squamous Cell Carcinoma

Practical Pearls

- For curettage and electrocoagulation of malignant tumors, a semi-sharp curette can be used. An aggressive curettage is performed in multiple directions, aiming to find and remove small extensions of the tumor into the surrounding skin. Care should be taken when curetting the surrounding skin in an elderly patient with friable skin.

- After curettage, the curetted wound bed is coagulated. Electrofulguration provides superficial coagulation. The surgeon continues fulgurating until hemostasis is achieved. An aggressive fulguration using high power and moving the electrode very slowly on the skin will provide a deeper coagulation. Using the flat side of a knife-shaped electrode as a brush can make the fulguration much faster and more homogenous compared with using the sharp tip of the electrode. After fulguration, the superficial coagulated tissue may be removed with a curette and the procedure may be repeated.
- Performing contact coagulation (instead of fulguration) after the first curettage can provide deeper coagulation with no need for repeating curettage. In addition to providing a wider zone of tissue destruction, contact coagulation has the added benefits of being associated with much less smoke as well as being more reliable and effective in providing hemostasis than fulguration.
- Injecting saline or lidocaine into the superficial subcutaneous plane under the tumor elevates the tumor and isolates it from the deeper structures, reducing the risk of damage to nerves, vessels, or cartilage during deep coagulation.

Curettage and electrocoagulation for BCC and cSCC has shown different cure rates in different studies. The main reasons for the inconsistent outcome data for curettage and electrocoagulation can be a lack of standardization of curettage as well as a lack of clear definitions of electrosurgical terms in the literature. Different surgeons may perform curettage or electrosurgical procedures differently. Some surgeons use a curette only to gently debulk the tumor, while others perform a more aggressive curette, trying to remove all of the tumoral tissue [31, 61]. Many surgeons perform electrofulguration, while others may perform a deeper desiccation after curettage. Since a gentle fulguration just to the point of hemostasis may provide a coagulation depth around one-tenth of the depth of true deep desiccation, the recurrence rate of the procedures with electrofulguration may be higher than those with deeper desiccation [2, 43]. On the other hand, an effective curettage and electrocoagulation performed by an experienced surgeon can have a success rate comparable to or even higher than excision [62].

5.4.6.1 Curettage

A more aggressive curettage can improve the cure rate of curettage and electrocoagulation for skin cancer. The surgeons who use a curette gently to debulk the tumor may have a lower cure rate than the ones who use the curette to aggressively scrape and remove all of the friable tumoral tissues and maybe a thin layer of the surrounding skin.

An aggressive curettage is performed using a semi-sharp curette in multiple directions, aiming to find and remove all extensions of the tumor. Some surgeons may use a larger curette (4 or 5 mm) first to remove most of the tumoral tissue and then a smaller curette (2 or 2.5 mm) to look for small extensions of the tumor. After the removal of tumoral tissue, some surgeons may use a sharp curette to remove a thin layer of the normal tissue on the wound bed that may have microscopic extensions of the tumor. In experienced hands, an aggressive curettage alone can provide a cure rate comparable to curettage and electrocoagulation in both BCC and cSCC. A retrospective cohort of 1853 total lesions treated with curettage showed a 5-year recurrence rate of 2.41% for BCCs and 4.52% for cSCCs [63–65]. Using electrocoagulation after a semi-sharp curettage can provide hemostasis as well as destruction of a margin of surrounding tissue; therefore, there is no need for using a sharp curette. One disadvantage of electrocoagulation is its potential risks to patients with implanted electronic devices. An aggressive curettage followed by chemical cautery or hot iron electrocautery is an acceptable alternative in patients with contraindications for high-frequency electrosurgery.

If using a disposable ring-shaped curette, the back of the ring can be used as a blunt or semi-sharp curette. The sharp edge of the curette can also be scraped against a hard object (e.g., a scalpel) to make it semi-sharp.

When working on aged and sun-damaged friable skin, a blunt curette may be a safer choice for removing tumoral tissue while avoiding overtreatment or accidental tearing of the skin. On the other hand, when working on an anatomic area with terminal hairs, a sharp curette may be the best choice to have the job done.

5.4.6.2 Electrocoagulation After Curettage

Electrocoagulation after curettage can be performed using fulguration or contact coagulation.

Electrofulguration typically provides a thin layer of coagulation. To provide a deeper depth of destruction, this thin coagulated layer can be removed using another pass of curettage followed by another pass of fulguration. Alternatively, a more aggressive fulguration or contact coagulation can be used to provide a thicker layer of coagulation in one pass that may not need to be curetted again.

Electrofulguration

One of the most performed methods of electrocoagulation after curettage is touching the base of the wound with the electrode while the generator is already active. This method produces sparks and smoke and provides fulguration with relatively superficial coagulation. The surgeon continues fulgurating until hemostasis is achieved. Continuing fulguration after hemostasis will increase the depth of coagulation.

Electrofulguration can be performed using a fine-tip electrode such as the tip of a knife-shaped electrode. A fine-tip electrode can focus the sprayed current on a small target. For fulgurating a larger target, a large-tip electrode such as the flat side of a knife-shaped electrode is preferred. A large-tip fulgurating electrode can provide more homogenous hemostasis and coagulation on the target in a shorter time. Fulguration using a large-tip electrode needs a relatively higher output power to be dialed on the electrosurgical generator front panel. If the tissue surface is not flat, the electrode needs to be pressed against it firmly to have a good "contact" and provide a homogenous fulguration on all the target areas. If the electrode sticks to the tissue and stops sparking, a higher power needs to be dialed, or the electrode needs to be pressed less firmly.

Electrofulguration using a large-tip electrode is probably the easiest and fastest method of coagulation of the wound bed after curettage. In experienced hands, it can provide an acceptable hemostasis homogenously with relatively superficial coagulation. Again, continuing fulguration after hemostasis can provide a deeper coagulation.

Contact Coagulation

Contact coagulation is an alternative to fulguration for providing a deeper coagulation (Table 5.3). A true desiccation can provide coagulation as deep as 5 mm or more. This deep margin on and around the wound bed can be associated with a higher cure rate than when performing a superficial fulguration [2]. In addition to providing a wider zone of tissue destruction and better hemostasis, contact coagulation is associated with much less smoke and, theoretically, less risk of infection spread through evaporated tissue particles than fulguration [1]. One limitation of contact coagulation is that the depth of tissue destruction is not visible. If the surgeon prefers not to coagulate the whole dermis, multiple passes of curettage and fulguration may give the surgeon better control over the depth of destruction.

When there is significant bleeding from a wound bed, using a small-tip electrode or a low-power setting may not work. Using a large-tip electrode and using higher power may be more effective for hemostasis on a severely bleeding scalp wound.

Table 5.3 Different methods of coagulation used on wound bed after curettage of skin lesions

	Depth of coagulation	Electrode size	Power setting	Pros	Cons
Fulguration	+	Small tip	Low	Fast and easy	Smoke. Homogenous hemostasis is hard to achieve
	++	Large tip	High	Fast and easy	Smoke
Contact coagulation	++	Small tip (a small ball-shaped electrode; the edge of a knife-shaped electrode can be used as a brush)	The power should be enough to provide hemostasis with a fast movement of the electrode on the tissue surface	No smoke	Homogenous hemostasis is hard to achieve. Needs experience
	+++	Large tip (a ball-shaped electrode; flat side of a knife-shaped electrode can move parallel to its long axis)	The power should be enough to provide hemostasis with a fast movement of the electrode on the tissue surface	Fast and easy. No smoke	Needs experience
	++++	Large tip (a ball-shaped electrode; flat side of a knife-shaped electrode can be used as a brush)	The power should be enough to provide desiccation with a fast movement of the electrode on the tissue surface	Fast and easy	Tissue boiling and occasional fulguration increases the chance of airborne infections but not as high as fulguration
	+++++	Large tip (a ball-shaped electrode; flat side of a knife-shaped electrode can be used as a brush)	The power should be enough to provide desiccation with a slow movement of the electrode on the tissue surface	The most effective hemostasis and highest cancer cure rate	Slow. The depth of injury can be too deep. Tissue boiling and occasional fulguration increases the chance of airborne infections

5.5 Electrosurgery in the Treatment of Benign Superficial Skin Lesions

Benign epidermal lesions such as seborrheic keratoses can be treated by selective coagulation of the epidermis and papillary dermis while preserving the reticular dermis intact to avoid scar formation.

Upon a mild thermal coagulation, the epidermis and papillary dermis turn into a soft material (liquefaction) that can be easily wiped off the skin surface [1]. In contrast, the reticular dermis contracts and maintains its solidity and durability after coagulation and cannot be wiped off [66]. This phenomenon helps the surgeon differentiate between papillary dermis and reticular dermis, potentially avoiding unnecessary deep injuries and scar formation.

In order to perform very superficial coagulation of the epidermis and papillary dermis, a needle-shaped electrode can be used in the contact method. The power should be low but enough to provide liquefaction of the epidermis with a fast movement of the electrode on the target. A very slow heating process should be avoided because it increases the chance of heat conduction and deep injury. Using high-voltage interrupted currents (fulguration or coagulation mode) may cause large spark formation when the electrode loses contact with the tissue and, therefore, should be avoided. A continuous current (cutting mode) can be a good choice if the mode can be dialed to a very low power.

A very dry thick stratum corneum (superficial dead layer of the epidermis) may show a high electrical resistance and may not pass electrosurgical currents effectively. Soaking the epidermis with water or saline makes coagulation and liquefaction of the epidermis easier to achieve.

Spark formation that occurs at the time of desiccation means overtreatment and the occurrence of deeper injury. Desiccation and spark formation should be avoided by reducing voltage, power, and/or contact time.

When liquefaction of the epidermis is achieved, the soft coagulated materials can be wiped off or scraped off using the active electrode, and the process can be repeated if needed.

Using the tip of a needle-shaped electrode in contact mode may be slow and not practical for larger epidermal lesions. Fulguration is an alternative method of providing superficial coagulation for larger lesions. The power should be enough to provide coagulation of the epidermis with a fast movement of the electrode on the target.

Seborrheic Keratosis

Seborrheic keratoses are usually treated using cryotherapy. Since cryotherapy is associated with a higher risk of dyspigmentation in dark skins, electrocoagulation may be used as an alternative for smaller seborrheic keratoses on darker skins.

Common Warts or Genital Warts

Although electrocautery is an available therapeutic option for viral warts, it is not commonly used because of concern for viral transmission through the explosion of infected cells and smoke. The use of a smoke evacuator may reduce, but may not eliminate, the risk of viral transmission. If safer therapeutic options such as cryosurgery are not available or not indicated, a very gentle electrocoagulation (liquefaction) of the epidermis, similar to the method described for seborrheic keratosis, can be used while trying to avoid any explosion or spark formation. After wiping off the coagulated epidermis, the reticular dermis at the base of the wart can be treated using Drysol (aluminum chloride in alcohol), silver nitrate cautery, or low concentration of trichloroacetic acid, in order to provide hemostasis and theoretically to kill the remaining viruses or infected cells.

Facial Plane Warts

Multiple facial plane warts are sometimes a therapeutic challenge. The author's experience is that a very superficial contact coagulation similar to the method explained for common warts can provide an acceptable clearance rate with a low risk of scar formation on the face. Again, the author uses Drysol or a low concentration of trichloroacetic acid on the surgical site after wiping off the coagulated epidermis. The risk of scar formation using this method is higher on the lips and in children before puberty. The use of a smoke evacuator is strongly recommended.

Sebaceous Hyperplasia

Sebaceous hyperplasia is a common benign small papular lesion on the face in middle-aged or elderly patients. Although it is asymptomatic and benign, it may cause cosmetic concerns in some people. The enlarged sebaceous glands are mainly in the superficial dermis. Similar to epidermis, sebaceous glands turn into a soft material (liquefaction) when coagulated.

Treatment of sebaceous hyperplasia with electrosurgery is usually very easy with good cosmetic outcomes. A needle-shaped electrode can be used in the same way as described for seborrheic keratosis. The difference is that sebaceous hyperplasia is in the superficial dermis rather than on top of it.

Syringoma

Syringoma is a common cosmetic problem presenting multiple small flat papules on the lower eyelids. The abnormal eccrine glands usually extend into the thin reticular dermis, and therefore any destructive measures aiming at removing these glands will result in minimal scar. Because the syringoma itself is not a major cosmetic issue, the scar that may remain at the site of surgery may not be more acceptable to the patient than the syringoma itself. The author usually treats one or two lesions and lets the patient decide after a few months if he or she wants to proceed to the treatment of the other lesions. The treatment method is the same as for sebaceous hyperplasia.

Milium

Milia are small superficial white keratin-filled cysts more commonly found on the face and around the eyelids. They are more common in neonates and may be seen after reepithelialization of a second-degree wound. Most milia resolve spontaneously after the roof of the cyst opens and the contents come out. If treatment is needed for cosmetic reasons, the roof of the cyst can be cut using a surgical knife or a needle. The contents can be extracted at the time of the procedure, or if the cut on the roof is long enough, they may come out later spontaneously.

Cutting the roof of the lesions using a sharp tool may be slow and time-consuming if there are multiple milia. A sharp needle-shaped electrosurgical electrode in cutting mode can cut the roof of a milium in less than a second. The power output should be at the minimum level that enables the surgeon to cut briskly. Using higher power is associated with more pain if anesthesia has not been applied. The lesion can be left alone after the cut for the content to come out spontaneously.

Xanthelasma

Xanthelasmas are yellowish papules and plaques most commonly found on periorbital skin. Histopathologically, there is an accumulation of lipid deposits within large, pale, fat-laden histiocytes in the dermis.

Xanthelasma can be excised or treated using different destructive techniques, including electrosurgery.

Electrofulguration with or without curettage can be used for larger xanthelasmas. Smaller xanthomas can be treated using a needle-shaped electrode in contact mode, similar to the method described above for sebaceous hyperplasia. Removal of xanthelasma using destructive methods usually leaves some degree of scarring, which can be acceptable to most patients.

Small Melanocytic Nevus

Electrosurgery is an alternative to punch excision for the treatment of small melanocytic nevi. The major advantage of electrosurgery over punch excision is that, during electrosurgery, the pigmented tissue can be selectively coagulated and scraped off without removing normal underlying tissue. Therefore, the risk for scar formation can potentially be less when the pigmented cells do not involve a deeper dermis.

The major disadvantages of electrosurgery for the treatment of melanocytic nevus are the inability to send tissue for histopathologic examination and a higher risk of recurrence compared with excision. Recurrence of the nevus is relatively common even if all the pigmented tissue is removed during electrosurgery. The recurrent pigmented nevus is usually not round or symmetrical and may clinically and histopathologically imitate malignant melanoma. If the primary lesion has not been sent for histopathological exam, a recurrent nevus may be labeled as malignant melanoma and may lead to unnecessary radical surgery.

There has always been a concern about the possibility of malignant transformation of a melanocytic nevus after thermal or physical trauma. This possibility has neither been proven nor unequivocally refuted. Most of the published studies on the use of laser or electrosurgery for melanocytic nevi did not show any evidence of malignant transformation. Pusey, Templeton, and Fowlkes reported no malignancy developing in any pigmented or nonpigmented nevi removed by them for cosmetic reasons over 105 combined work years [15, 67]. Nor were Walton and Cox [68] or Slaughter [69] able to find any authenticated instance of a benign nevus becoming malignant after incomplete removal with electrosurgery, cautery, or excision.

Walton and associates found no evidence of malignant change following the electrodesiccation of 467 pigmented nevi [70]. In a survey of 201 dermatologists with an estimated total nevi removal series of 1.65 million, Shaw found that 50.4% of them used some form of electrosurgery and 19.6% some other nonsurgical method, at least 90% of the time [67].

The easiest way to remove a melanocytic nevus using electrosurgery is to use a very sharp-tip electrode. Using a low-power cutting current, the pigmented tissue can be coagulated and scraped off using the same electrode. If the available electrodes are not sharp, the coagulated tissue can be scraped off using another tool such as a scalpel or a curette.

Telangiectasia

Telangiectasias are dilated superficial small blood vessels visible as red lines on the skin. Telangiectasias are located in the superficial dermis and should be differentiated from varicose veins, which are larger and located under the dermis in the subcutaneous tissue.

Treatment of telangiectasia involves the destruction of its lumen. Very thin superficial vessels are usually treated using vascular lasers. If there are a few telangiectasias, they can be treated one by one using an ablative laser or electrocoagulation performed on multiple spots along their course. Obliteration of the lumen of the vessel at multiple spots along its path will result in the resolution of the telangiectasia.

Spider Angioma

Spider angiomata are telangiectasia with a central feeding arteriole and some radiating telangiectatic vessels in the shape of spider legs. In order to treat a spider angioma, the central arteriole needs to be obliterated.

To perform a very gentle electrocoagulation of a spot along the course of a telangiectasia or on the central feeding arteriole of a spider angioma, a semi-sharp needle-shaped electrode is used with a relatively low-power setting in coagulation mode. Before activating the electrode, the tip of the needle is pressed on the target to force the blood out of the vessel lumen. If the electrode is too sharp, it may puncture the epidermis. The resulting bleeding will interfere with a gentle electrocoagulation. While the electrode is in contact with the skin, the generator is activated for less than 1 second. This short pulse should be able to coagulate the target and obliterate the vessel. If the energy is not enough to coagulate the target, the power setting or activation time may be increased. If the needle punctures the skin but fails to coagulate and obliterate the vessel, the procedure can be repeated at a nearby spot. Using a lower-power setting and keeping the activated electrode in contact with the target for a longer time provides deeper coagulation with less chance of cutting the skin. Deeper coagulation provides a higher cure rate at the cost of a higher risk of a pitted scar.

Radiating vessels of a spider angioma may not fill if the central arteriole is destroyed. Incompletely destroyed lesions may recur.

Treatment of larger telangiectasias can be performed using endovascular techniques used for varicose veins, such as sclerotherapy, endovascular lasers, or endovascular electrocoagulation electrodes (commonly known as radiofrequency probes).

For endovascular electrocoagulation, a very thin needle electrode, such as an epilation electrode or a 30-gauge needle, can be inserted in the target vessel. The proximal part of the needle can be insulated to prevent damage to the epidermis at the entrance point. A needle electrode adapter or epilation pen can be used for this purpose.

Cherry Angiomas

Cherry angiomas are benign small red spots with no malignant potential. If the patient requests treatment for cosmetic reasons, electrosurgery is probably the preferred option because it is relatively easy with good cosmetic outcomes. The method of treatment is the same as for sebaceous hyperplasia. Larger cherry angiomas may be shaved off first using a scalpel or a curette and then treated using electrocoagulation of the base. The skin may need to be pinched at the time of the procedure to stop bleeding (Fig. 5.8).

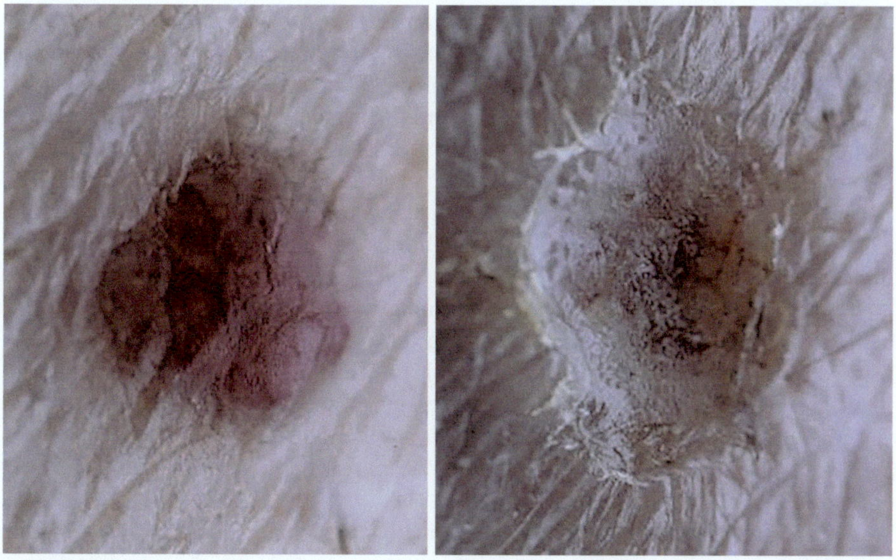

Fig. 5.8 A small (3-mm) cherry angioma on a knee treated with electrocoagulation. The sharp tip of a knife-shaped electrode and a very-low-power continuous current (cutting mode) were used. The superficial layer of the angioma was coagulated and scraped off using the active electrode. The process was repeated until all the vascular tissue was removed. The lesion was entirely in the papillary dermis. The pain was tolerable; therefore, no anesthesia was used. The plan was to pinch the area to prevent bleeding; however, there was no bleeding. The photo on the right shows the lesion immediately after the procedure

Pyogenic Granuloma

A pyogenic granuloma is an acquired benign proliferation of capillary blood vessels of the skin and mucous membranes. The name is a misnomer as it is a form of lobular capillary hemangioma, not a granuloma, and not due to infection. Pyogenic granuloma usually presents as a dome-shaped red papule made of friable vascular tissue that may extend into the deep dermis.

Curettage and electrosurgery is probably the preferred treatment for pyogenic granulomas; however, curettage may be associated with some bleeding [29]. To prevent excessive bleeding, the base of the lesion can be infiltrated with a solution of lidocaine plus epinephrine, if appropriate. After waiting for a few minutes for epinephrine to provide vasoconstriction, the exophytic portion of the lesion is shaved off with a scalpel or a sharp, large curette and sent for histopathological examination. All the remaining friable abnormal tissue is removed using a semi-sharp curette.

Once the bulk of the lesion is removed, the surgeon should apply pressure around the surgical site to stop bleeding. Then, the base of the wound will be treated using electrofulguration or very gentle contact coagulation to destroy a thin layer of the surface and achieve hemostasis.

Rhinophyma

Rhinophyma is a slowly progressive, disfiguring disorder of the nose that represents the end stage of rosacea, a relatively common centrofacial dermatosis. Chronic uncontrolled rosacea causes inflammation and edema in the skin that leads to connective tissue and sebaceous gland hypertrophy and thickening of the dermis, mainly at the level of the papillary dermis. Surgical treatment of rhinophyma includes the removal of hypertrophic tissue while saving the deeper reticular dermis to prevent scar formation.

The reticular dermis of the nose has a high density of epidermal appendages. Therefore, partial-thickness wounds and burns are less likely to cause scars in this area.

The hyperplastic papillary dermis, including sebaceous glands, can be shaved using a scalpel or removed using dermabrasion or ablative lasers. An advantage of using electrosurgery over a scalpel is that it is easier to differentiate between the papillary and reticular dermis and, therefore, easier to avoid scar formation when performing electrosurgery. Instant hemostasis is another advantage of electrosurgery.

Removal of the hyperplastic tissue can be performed using electrofulguration, contact coagulation, or loop electrosection.

A thin layer of tissue can be coagulated (liquefied) using fulguration or contact coagulation and wiped off. The procedure can be repeated until the reticular dermis is reached, which cannot be liquefied using heat.

For larger masses, a loop electrode made of a very thin wire can be used to cut and remove larger masses of tissue. The procedure can be started using a relatively low output power, trying to cut and remove the tissue through liquefaction rather than through tissue explosion and classical electrosection. An experienced surgeon may be able to feel the change in consistency and tissue response to electrosection when the electrode enters the denser reticular dermis. However, this is not always the case, and loop electrosection may work as a scalpel, especially when using a relatively high output power for a classical loop electrosection. For the removal of tissues with more fibrotic stroma, liquefaction may never happen, and a classical loop electrosection may be the only effective method.

The surgeon should exercise a conservative approach to shaping the nose. Although some degree of scar formation is acceptable after removing large masses of rhinophyma from an elderly patient's nose, undertreatment is easier to correct than dealing with a nonhealing wound or a contracting scar secondary to overtreatment.

Fibrous rhinophyma is a less common variant of rhinophyma characterized histologically by telangiectasia, diffuse dermal fibrosis with abundant mucin, and a virtual absence of pilosebaceous structures [71]. This variant is harder to treat using ablative lasers or electrosurgery, compared with the common variant. Scalpel sculpturing or loop electrosection can be performed by an experienced surgeon with acceptable results.

Skin Tags

Skin tags can be grabbed and pulled up using forceps and then cut using a scalpel, scissors, or electrosection. Electrosection has the advantage of providing hemostasis at the time of cutting and makes the procedure much faster when there are multiple lesions treated. Figure 5.9 shows how to reduce the risk of scar formation when removing a skin tag using an electrosection.

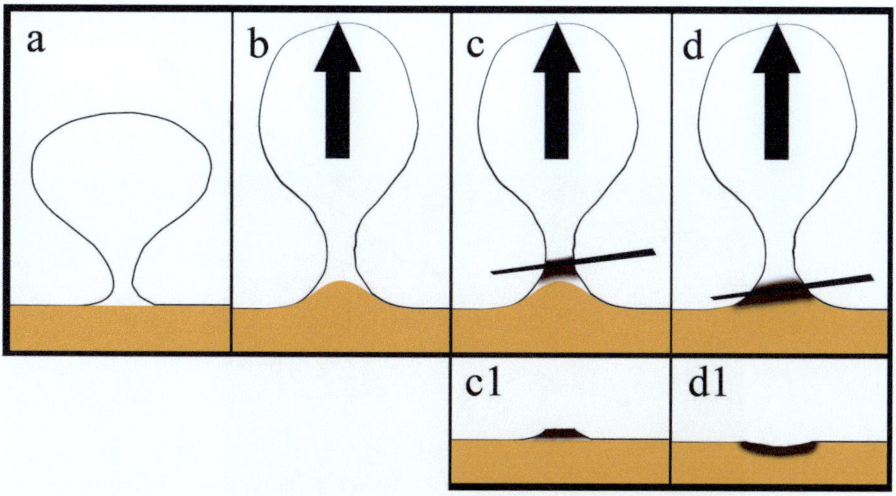

Fig. 5.9 Removing a skin tag using electrosection. (**a**, **b**) The skin tag is grabbed and pulled away from the skin using forceps. (**c**) Pulling the skin tag up pulls the underlying dermis up as well. The cut should be made high enough to avoid the dermis. (**d**) Cutting too close to the skin may cause a deep injury and scar

An alternative method for treating a small skin tag with a narrow stalk is grabbing the skin tag using metallic forceps, twisting the skin tag minimally to make the stalk even narrower, and then touching the active electrode to the forceps. The electrosurgical current enters the tag and burns the narrow stalk when flowing to the patient's body. The skin tag with a burned stalk can be left to fall off itself. This method may not be preferred when dealing with a large skin tag, because of the risk of infection if a larger necrotic mass is left on the skin.

5.6 Electrosurgery for Treatment of Deep Dermal or Subcutaneous Targets Using Penetrating Proximally Insulated Electrodes

Electrocoagulation of a variety of tumors in internal organs has been performed using penetrating proximally insulated electrodes [72, 73]. Recently, this approach has been used for the treatment of the deeper component of infantile hemangioma of the skin (Fig. 5.10) [74].

Complete coagulation of a large subcutaneous mass may cause severe local or even systemic inflammation. To avoid a severe inflammatory reaction, treatment can be performed in multiple sessions, a few weeks apart. If treatment is for cosmetic reasons, the sessions may be spaced months apart to let inflammation resolve completely and scar tissue mature in order to avoid overtreatment.

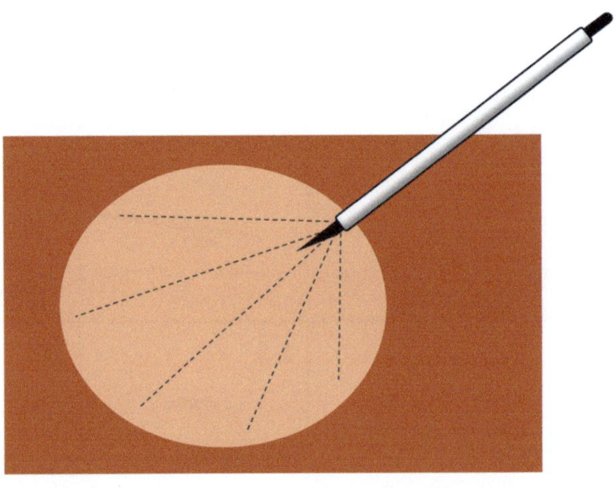

Fig. 5.10 Transcutaneous electrocoagulation of subcutaneous targets. Electrosurgical current can be delivered to a subcutaneous target using a penetrating electrode. Insulation of the proximal parts of the electrode protects the superficial tissue from thermal damage. To coagulate a large mass, the electrode can move back and forth in different directions in the target
Dotted lines show the paths of movement of the electrode in the target

Endovascular thermal ablation of varicose veins is a less invasive alternative to traditional surgery. In this method, a long flexible electrosurgical electrode with insulation on the proximal parts enters the veins and coagulates the internal lumen. Compared to surgery, this approach provides the same efficacy with less postoperative morbidity and a lower rate of adverse events [75–77].

5.7 Electrosurgical Currents in Aesthetic Medicine and Skin Rejuvenation

High-frequency electrical currents (radiofrequency or RF technology) have been used for the treatment of cellulite, acne scars, inflammatory acne, and nonablative tightening of skin to improve laxity and reduce wrinkles [78–85].

Most of the devices marketed for skin rejuvenation use one or more electrodes to deliver the current to the epidermal surface. The manufacturers of some of those devices claim that the application of radiofrequency energy (a fancy name for high-frequency alternating electrical currents) to the skin causes heating of dermal tissue with subsequent remodeling of collagen fibers and neocollagenesis that can lead to skin tightening and rejuvenation [85, 86]. None of the devices that deliver the current to the epidermal surface has gained much attention in scientific literature, and there is a paucity of well-conducted randomized trials supporting their efficacy [86]. In contrast with those devices, fractional radiofrequency microneedling systems use penetrating electrodes to deliver the electrical currents directly into the deeper dermis (Fig. 5.11). Multi-electrode pins of these devices provide heating of the areas in direct contact with penetrating electrodes, leaving intact or only slightly affected zones in the dermis between the targeted areas. The preserved tissue serves as a pool of cells that promote rapid wound healing [87–92].

Depending on the technology used, when an electrode of a fractional radiofrequency device enters the skin, the maximum heating effect can be around the tip of the electrode in the dermis [93]. This phenomenon can preserve the epidermis during dermal heating and reduce the risk of post-procedural side effects, including post-inflammatory dyspigmentation. By insulating the proximal parts of the penetrating electrode, the epidermis can be saved even better during heating of the dermis [74, 88]. In contrast to radiofrequency currents, laser-based fractional resurfacing produces greater tissue injury on the skin surface (epidermis) than in the deep dermis and, as a result, may cause more post-procedural side effects [94]. However, to our knowledge, there is no clinical trial comparing these modalities.

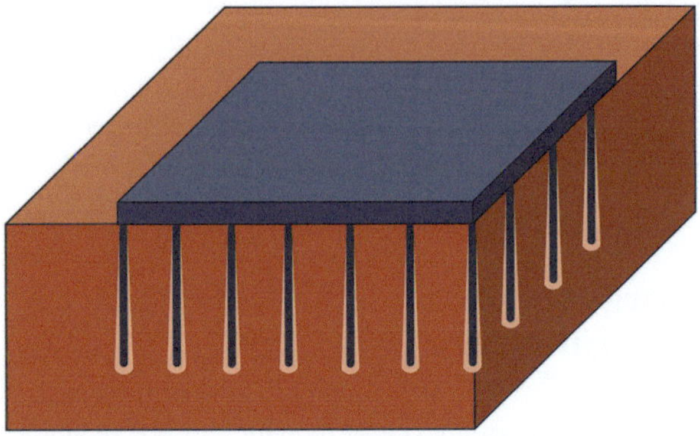

Fig. 5.11 The active electrode of a fractional radiofrequency microneedling device has multiple small needles that enter the skin, deep into the dermis. The part of the electrode on top of the epidermis is insulated and does not pass significant energy directly to the epidermis. When a high-frequency (radiofrequency) electrical current passes through the electrode and those needles, it causes heating with potential coagulation of the areas in contact with the penetrating electrodes (light-brown areas around the needles). The maximum heating effect of the electrode will be around the tip of the needles in deeper tissue. The reason is that charged particles of the same polarity (positive versus negative) in any object tend to be as far apart as possible, rather than being homogeneously distributed. Therefore, the net electric charge of the electrode resides more on its extremities and tip of the needles than along their shaft

5.8 Practicing Electrosurgery in a Lab

Practicing electrosurgery in a lab can help with having some hands-on experience and building confidence. The most widely used substrate for practicing electrosurgery is the banana. However, animal liver tissue is preferred and strongly recommended over bananas because it is more similar to human tissues. The liver changes color to light brown upon exposure to heat; so, the surgeon can see the depth of coagulation during or after the procedure.

Trainees can try cutting the tissue with different knives or a thin wire. They can use different waveforms at different power settings and different speeds and compare the thickness of coagulated tissue on the incision walls. Finding the lowest power setting that can enable the electrode to cut fast should be the goal. Cutting current can be tried to provide a clean cut, and blend or coagulation current to provide a blend cut.

Fulguration can be performed using different waveforms at different power settings. Trainees can use the tip of a knife-shaped electrode for smaller areas or the flat side of the electrode as a large brush for larger areas. Practicing fulguration using the flat side of a knife-shaped electrode while using a high-power setting is strongly recommended. This is a very useful procedure that some dermatologists may be hesitant to try on their patients. If the electrode sticks to the tissue, the power should be increased. Trainees can observe the superficial depth of coagulation associated with fast fulguration, even when high power is used. Then, they can practice slow fulguration by keeping the active sparking electrode on a specific area for a few seconds. After practicing different methods, they can cut the treated tissue using a scalpel and compare the depth of coagulation associated with different methods of fulguration and also with contact coagulation.

A fine-tip electrode can be used at a low-power setting for superficial contact coagulation of smaller areas.

A large-tip electrode can be used for deep contact coagulation or desiccation of larger targets. Different power settings can be tried. The flat side of a knife-shaped electrode can touch tissue, and then the electrode can be moved on the tissue surface in a direction parallel to the long axis of the electrode at a speed enough to leave a track of coagulated tissue behind. If the electrode sticks to the tissue, the tissue can be moistened, or a faster movement of the electrode on the tissue can be tried. Spot treatment methods can also be tried as an alternative.

If the electrosurgical generator is earth-referenced, all the procedures can be tried with or without using a return electrode. Using a return electrode increases the available power at the electrode–tissue interface at any dialed setting.

5.9 Practical Differences Between Different Electrosurgical Units

Electrosurgical units have different output power and output frequencies and can provide different modes. When choosing a generator for a dermatology practice, we should consider whether we need it for a surgical room or for an office exam room, how much maximum power we may need, if the device can provide very low output power for very superficial coagulation, and if it is earth-referenced or isolated. The choice of the unit depends on the surgical setting and the desired applications (Table 5.4).

Some electrosurgical units show an index named "crest factor," which is the ratio of peak voltage to average voltage of their output currents. If there is only one crest factor reported, it is usually for their continuous cutting current. A generator with a lower crest factor in its cutting mode can provide cleaner cuts with less coagulation on the incision walls and less hemostasis in pure cutting mode. However, since coagulation on the incision walls depends on many factors, including the thickness of the electrode used, the power setting, and the speed of movement of the electrode, minor changes in crest factor may not change the quality of the cut significantly. On the other hand, electrosection is used instead of a scalpel when hemostasis is needed. Therefore, a very low crest factor may not be needed and, therefore, may not be a major advantage of an electrosurgical unit. A generator with a higher crest factor and a higher peak voltage in its fulguration mode can provide larger sparks for easier fulguration compared with its competitors. This advantage helps mainly when using a small electrode for fulgurating a large surface area. An experienced

Table 5.4 The choice of the electrosurgical unit based on the surgical setting

Setting and indications	Commonly used devices	Advantages	Disadvantages
Major surgeries and endoscopic (urologic) procedures in operating rooms	High power (usually 200–400 watt output power), isolated generators	May have more available modes and flexibility for procedures needing high power	Expensive. Some high-power devices may lack the ability to provide a very low output power for very superficial minor destruction. Automatic power adjustment mode is not the best option for dermatologic surgeries
Minor dermatologic procedures on conscious patients	Low power (usually around 40–100 watt output power), earth-referenced units	More cost-effective and convenient to use	May have fewer available modes and flexibility
Most dermatologic procedures	Medium power (usually around 70–200 watt output power), earth-referenced or isolated units Fulguration mode should be able to provide large sparks Cutting mode should have the option to be dialed to a very low power for contact coagulation of small epidermal lesions	One device for all dermatologic electrosurgical procedures	Isolated units may be less convenient to use than earth-referenced units

surgeon who knows how to use a large electrode as a large brush may not need a very high voltage current, so it may not be an advantage.

Most available electrosurgical units in the market have an output frequency of 0.3–5 MHz. There is no strong evidence demonstrating any relation between the frequency of electrosurgical currents and their surgical effects on tissue. One in vitro study comparing electrosurgical currents at different frequencies did not find any relation between the frequency of electrosurgical currents and the depth or pattern of electrocoagulation [3]. A few studies are available that favor some frequencies; however, these studies can be criticized because of poor study methods [95].

Most conventional electrosurgical generators used in dermatologic surgery use a *constant voltage output* system. In these generators, voltage is the output variable that is adjusted on the display panel. The output power that is delivered to the target depends not only on the voltage of the device that is dialed on the display but also on the resistance at the electrode–tissue interface. The dial setting for control of voltage in most older units was an arbitrary number setting (e.g., 1–10). More recent *constant voltage* generators are supplemented with a dial setting with a display calibrated in watts. However, like the older devices, voltage is the output variable that is adjusted using this dial panel, not power. The indicated "power" number that is dialed actually refers to the maximum power that can be delivered at that voltage setting and, again, is dependent on the resistance at the electrode–tissue interface. This type of display has the advantage of allowing some degree of comparison to be made between different units or modes.

References

1. Taheri A, Mansoori P, Sandoval LF, Feldman SR, Pearce D, Williford PM. Electrosurgery: part II. Technology, applications, and safety of electrosurgical devices. J Am Acad Dermatol. 2014;70(4):607.e1–12; quiz 619–20. https://doi.org/10.1016/j.jaad.2013.09.055. PubMed PMID: 24629362.
2. Taheri A, Green C, Mansoori P. Controlling depth of electrosurgery after curettage of skin tumors-an in vitro study. Int J Dermatol. 2019;58(12):1472–6. https://doi.org/10.1111/ijd.14631. PubMed PMID: 31531982.
3. Taheri A, Mansoori P, Bahrami N, Alinia H, Watkins CE, Feldman SR. How frequency of electrosurgical current and electrode size affect the depth of electrocoagulation. Dermatol Surg. 2016;42(2):197–202. https://doi.org/10.1097/DSS.0000000000000593. PubMed PMID: 26783688.
4. Taheri A, Mansoori P, Sandoval LF, Feldman SR, Pearce D, Williford PM. Electrosurgery: part I. Basics and principles. J Am Acad Dermatol. 2014;70(4):591.e1–14; quiz 605–6. https://doi.org/10.1016/j.jaad.2013.09.056. PubMed PMID: 24629361.
5. Kalkwarf KL, Krejci RF, Edison AR. A method to measure operating variables in electrosurgery. J Prosthet Dent. 1979;42(5):566–70. PubMed PMID: 290807.
6. Strock MS. The rationale for electrosurgery. Oral Surg Oral Med Oral Pathol. 1952;5(11):1166–72. PubMed PMID: 13003151.
7. Noble WH, McClatchey KD, Douglass GD. A histologic comparison of effects of electrosurgical resection using different electrodes. J Prosthet Dent. 1976;35(5):575–9. PubMed PMID: 1063874.
8. Aird LNF, Brown CJ. Systematic review and meta-analysis of electrocautery versus scalpel for surgical skin incisions. Am J Surg. 2012;204(2):216–21. https://doi.org/10.1016/j.amjsurg.2011.09.032. PubMed PMID: 22537473.
9. Kashkouli MB, Kaghazkanai R, Mirzaie AZ, Hashemi M, Parvaresh MM, Sasanii L. Clinicopathologic comparison of radiofrequency versus scalpel incision for upper blepharoplasty. Ophthalmic Plast Reconstr Surg. 2008;24(1537-2677 (Electronic)):450–3. https://doi.org/10.1097/IOP.0b013e31818acfce. PubMed PMID: 19033840.
10. Loh SA, Carlson GA, Chang EI, Huang E, Palanker D, Gurtner GC. Comparative healing of surgical incisions created by the PEAK PlasmaBlade, conventional electrosurgery, and a scalpel. Plast Reconstr Surg. 2009;124(1529-4242 (Electronic)):1849–59. https://doi.org/10.1097/PRS.0b013e3181bcee87. PubMed PMID: 19952641.
11. Silverman EB, Read RW, Boyle CR, Cooper R, Miller WW, McLaughlin RM. Histologic comparison of canine skin biopsies collected using monopolar electrosurgery, CO2 laser, radiowave radiosurgery, skin biopsy punch, and scalpel. Vet Surg. 2007;36(0161-3499 (Print)):50–6. https://doi.org/10.1111/j.1532-950X.2007.00234.x. PubMed PMID: 17214820.
12. Sinha UK, Gallagher LA. Effects of steel scalpel, ultrasonic scalpel, CO2 laser, and monopolar and bipolar electrosurgery on wound healing in guinea pig oral mucosa. Laryngoscope. 2003;113(0023-852X (Print)):228–36. https://doi.org/10.1097/00005537-200302000-00007. PubMed PMID: 12567074.

13. Matsumoto K, Suzuki H, Usami Y, Hattori M, Komoro T. Histological evaluation of artifacts in tongue tissue produced by the CO2 laser and the electrotome. Photomed Laser Surg. 2008;26(1557-8550 (Electronic)):573–7. https://doi.org/10.1089/pho.2007.2217. PubMed PMID: 19025408.
14. Mausberg R, Visser H, Aschoff T, Donath K, Kruger W. Histology of laser- and high-frequency-electrosurgical incisions in the palate of pigs. J Craniomaxillofac Surg. 1993;21(1010-5182 (Print)):130–2. PubMed PMID: 8491862.
15. Elliott JA. Electrosurgery. Its use in dermatology, with a review of its development and technologic aspects. Arch Dermatol. 1966;94(0003-987X (Print)):340–50. PubMed PMID: 4952822.
16. Revercomb CH, Stewart CE, Bux RC. Artifact from an electrosurgical ground pad. Am J Forensic Med Pathol. 1997;18(0195-7910 (Print)):293–4. PubMed PMID: 9290879.
17. Schoinohoriti OK, Chrysomali E, Iatrou I, Perrea D. Evaluation of lateral thermal damage and reepithelialization of incisional wounds created by CO(2)-laser, monopolar electrosurgery, and radiosurgery: a pilot study on porcine oral mucosa. Oral Surg Oral Med Oral Pathol Oral Radiol Endod. 2011;(1528-395X (Electronic)). https://doi.org/10.1016/j.tripleo.2011.06.016. PubMed PMID: 21906972.
18. Basterra J, Zapater E, Moreno R, Hernandez R. Electrosurgical endoscopic cordectomy with microdissection electrodes: a comparative study with CO2 laser. J Laryngol Otol. 2006;120(1748-5460 (Electronic)):661–4. https://doi.org/10.1017/S0022215106001368. PubMed PMID: 16719953.
19. Courey MS, Fomin D, Smith T, Huang S, Sanders D, Reinisch L. Histologic and physiologic effects of electrocautery, CO2 laser, and radiofrequency injury in the porcine soft palate. Laryngoscope. 1999;109(0023-852X (Print)):1316–9. https://doi.org/10.1097/00005537-199908000-00025. PubMed PMID: 10443841.
20. Schemmel M, Haefner HK, Selvaggi SM, Warren JS, Termin CS, Hurd WW. Comparison of the ultrasonic scalpel to CO2 laser and electrosurgery in terms of tissue injury and adhesion formation in a rabbit model. Fertil Steril. 1997;67(0015-0282 (Print)):382–6. https://doi.org/10.1016/S0015-0282(97)81926-7. PubMed PMID: 9022618.
21. Stelter K, de la Chaux R, Patscheider M, Olzowy B. Double-blind, randomised, controlled study of post-operative pain in children undergoing radiofrequency tonsillotomy versus laser tonsillotomy. J Laryngol Otol. 2010;124(1748-5460 (Electronic)):880–5. https://doi.org/10.1017/S0022215110000605. PubMed PMID: 20380764.
22. Zapater E, Frias S, Perez A, Basterra J. Comparative study on chronic tissue damage after cordectomies using either CO2 laser or microdissection electrodes. Head Neck. 2009;31(1097-0347 (Electronic)):1477–81. https://doi.org/10.1002/hed.21115. PubMed PMID: 19378326.
23. Ahmed I, Berth-Jones J, Charles-Holmes S, O'Callaghan CJ, Ilchyshyn A. Comparison of cryotherapy with curettage in the treatment of Bowen's disease: a prospective study. Br J Dermatol. 2000;143(4):759–66. https://doi.org/10.1046/j.1365-2133.2000.03772.x. PubMed PMID: 11069453.
24. Fournier S, Laroche A, Leblanc M, Bourgeault E, Ulrich Singbo MN, Turcotte S, et al. Prospective clinical trial comparing curettage and cryosurgery to curettage and electrodesiccation in the management of minimally invasive basal and squamous cell carcinomas. J Cutan Med Surg. 2020;24(6):596–600. https://doi.org/10.1177/1203475420943258. PubMed PMID: 32721237.
25. Buzina DS, Lipozencic J. Electrosurgery—have we forgotten it? Acta Dermatovenerol Croat. 2007;15(1330-027X (Print)):96–102. PubMed PMID: 17631790.
26. Liew SH. Unwanted body hair and its removal: a review. Dermatologic Surg. 1999;25(1076-0512 (Print)):431–9. PubMed PMID: 10469088.
27. Olsen EA. Methods of hair removal. J Am Acad Dermatol. 1999;40(0190-9622 (Print)):143–55. PubMed PMID: 10025738.
28. Wagner RF Jr, Tomich JM, Grande DJ. Electrolysis and thermolysis for permanent hair removal. J Am Acad Dermatol. 1985;12(0190-9622 (Print)):441–9. PubMed PMID: 3989007.

29. Ghodsi SZ, Raziei M, Taheri A, Karami M, Mansoori P, Farnaghi F. Comparison of cryotherapy and curettage for the treatment of pyogenic granuloma: a randomized trial. Br J Dermatol. 2006;154(4):671–5. https://doi.org/10.1111/j.1365-2133.2005.06923.x. PubMed PMID: 16536810.
30. Bichakjian C, Armstrong A, Baum C, Bordeaux JS, Brown M, Busam KJ, et al. Guidelines of care for the management of basal cell carcinoma. J Am Acad Dermatol. 2018;78(3):540–59. https://doi.org/10.1016/j.jaad.2017.10.006. PubMed PMID: 29331385.
31. Kopf AW, Bart RS, Schrager D, Lazar M, Popkin GL. Curettage-electrodesiccation treatment of basal cell carcinomas. Arch Dermatol. 1977;113(4):439–43. PubMed PMID: 848972.
32. Silverman MK, Kopf AW, Grin CM, Bart RS, Levenstein MJ. Recurrence rates of treated basal cell carcinomas. Part 2: curettage-electrodesiccation. J Dermatol Surg Oncol. 1991;17(9):720–6. PubMed PMID: 1820764.
33. Silverman MK, Kopf AW, Grin CM, Bart RS, Levenstein MJ. Recurrence rates of treated basal cell carcinomas. Part 1: overview. J Dermatol Surg Oncol. 1991;17(9):713–8. PubMed PMID: 1890243.
34. Silverman MK, Kopf AW, Bart RS, Grin CM, Levenstein MS. Recurrence rates of treated basal cell carcinomas. Part 3: surgical excision. J Dermatol Surg Oncol. 1992;18(6):471–6. PubMed PMID: 1592998.
35. Rodriguez-Vigil T, Vázquez-López F, Perez-Oliva N. Recurrence rates of primary basal cell carcinoma in facial risk areas treated with curettage and electrodesiccation. J Am Acad Dermatol. 2007;56(1):91–5. https://doi.org/10.1016/j.jaad.2006.07.007. PubMed PMID: 17190625.
36. Rodríguez-Vigil T, Vázquez-López F, Pérez-Oliva N. Efficacy of curettage-electrodesiccation for basal cell carcinoma in medium- and high-risk areas. Actas Dermosifiliogr. 2011;102(8):633–4. https://doi.org/10.1016/j.ad.2011.01.016. PubMed PMID: 21798484.
37. Blixt E, Nelsen D, Stratman E. Recurrence rates of aggressive histologic types of basal cell carcinoma after treatment with electrodesiccation and curettage alone. Dermatol Surg. 2013;39(5):719–25. https://doi.org/10.1111/dsu.12122. PubMed PMID: 23379543.
38. Werlinger KD, Upton G, Moore AY. Recurrence rates of primary nonmelanoma skin cancers treated by surgical excision compared to electrodesiccation-curettage in a private dermatological practice. Dermatol Surg. 2002;28(12):1138–42; discussion 1142. PubMed PMID: 12472494.
39. Reymann F. Treatment of basal cell carcinoma of the skin with curettage. II. A follow-up study. Arch Dermatol. 1973;108(4):528–31. PubMed PMID: 4745285.
40. Mitchell JC, Hardie M. Treatment of basal cell carcinoma by curettage and electrosurgery. Can Med Assoc J. 1965;93:349–52. PubMed PMID: 14339294; PubMed Central PMCID: PMC1928756.
41. Williamson GS, Jackson R. Treatment of basal cell carcinoma by electrodesiccation and curettage. Can Med Assoc J. 1962;86:855–62. PubMed PMID: 14007244; PubMed Central PMCID: PMC1849182.
42. Zwald F, Practice gaps. Immediate curettage and electrodessication following biopsy of suspected basal cell carcinoma at initial visit. JAMA Dermatol. 2013;149(8):981. https://doi.org/10.1001/jamadermatol.2013.4463. PubMed PMID: 23760606.
43. Edens BL, Bartlow GA, Haghighi P, Astarita RW, Davidson TM. Effectiveness of curettage and electrodesiccation in the removal of basal cell carcinoma. J Am Acad Dermatol. 1983;9(3):383–8. PubMed PMID: 6630599.
44. Walker P, Hill D. Surgical treatment of basal cell carcinomas using standard postoperative histological assessment. Australas J Dermatol. 2006;47(1):1–12. https://doi.org/10.1111/j.1440-0960.2006.00216.x. PubMed PMID: 16405477.
45. Marchac D, Papadopoulos O, Duport G. Curative and aesthetic results of surgical treatment of 138 basal-cell carcinomas. J Dermatol Surg Oncol. 1982;8(5):379–87. PubMed PMID: 7096764.
46. Griffiths RW, Suvarna SK, Stone J. Do basal cell carcinomas recur after complete conventional surgical excision? Br J Plast Surg. 2005;58(6):795–805. https://doi.org/10.1016/j.bjps.2005.02.010. PubMed PMID: 16086990.

47. Breuninger H, Dietz K. Prediction of subclinical tumor infiltration in basal cell carcinoma. J Dermatol Surg Oncol. 1991;17(7):574–8. PubMed PMID: 1860987.
48. Wolf DJ, Zitelli JA. Surgical margins for basal cell carcinoma. Arch Dermatol. 1987;123(3):340–4. PubMed PMID: 3813602.
49. Kimyai-Asadi A, Alam M, Goldberg LH, Peterson SR, Silapunt S, Jih MH. Efficacy of narrow-margin excision of well-demarcated primary facial basal cell carcinomas. J Am Acad Dermatol. 2005;53(3):464–8. https://doi.org/10.1016/j.jaad.2005.03.038. PubMed PMID: 16112354.
50. Rowe DE, Carroll RJ, Day CL. Prognostic factors for local recurrence, metastasis, and survival rates in squamous cell carcinoma of the skin, ear, and lip: implications for treatment modality selection. J Am Acad Dermatol. 1992;26(6):976–90. https://doi.org/10.1016/0190-9622(92)70144-5.
51. Lansbury L, Bath-Hextall F, Perkins W, Stanton W, Leonardi-Bee J. Interventions for non-metastatic squamous cell carcinoma of the skin: systematic review and pooled analysis of observational studies. BMJ. 2013;347:f6153. https://doi.org/10.1136/bmj.f6153. PubMed PMID: 24191270.
52. Honeycutt WM, Jansen GT. Treatment of squamous cell carcinoma of the skin. Arch Dermatol. 1973;108(5):670–2. PubMed PMID: 4750203.
53. Reschly MJ, Shenefelt PD. Controversies in skin surgery: electrodessication and curettage versus excision for low-risk, small, well-differentiated squamous cell carcinomas. J Drugs Dermatol. 2010;9(7):773–6. PubMed PMID: 20677531.
54. Kauvar ANB, Arpey CJ, Hruza G, Olbricht SM, Bennett R. Consensus for nonmelanoma skin cancer treatment, part II: squamous cell carcinoma, including a cost analysis of treatment methods. Dermatologic Surg. 2015;41(11):1214–40. https://doi.org/10.1097/DSS.0000000000000478.
55. Freeman RG, Knox JM, Heaton CL. The treatment of skin cancer. A statistical study of 1,341 skin tumors comparing results obtained with irradiation, surgery, and curettage followed by electrodesiccation. Cancer. 1964;17:535–8. https://doi.org/10.1002/1097-0142(196404)17:4<535::aid-cncr2820170415>3.0.co;2-p. PubMed PMID: 14136537.
56. Alam M, Armstrong A, Baum C, Bordeaux JS, Brown M, Busam KJ, et al. Guidelines of care for the management of cutaneous squamous cell carcinoma. J Am Acad Dermatol. 2018;78(3):560–78. https://doi.org/10.1016/j.jaad.2017.10.007.
57. Matsumoto AJ, Schmitt AR, Skelley LM, Baum CL. Factors influencing squamous cell carcinoma in situ recurrence and implications for treatment choice. Dermatologic Surg. 2018;44(5):613–20. https://doi.org/10.1097/DSS.0000000000001400.
58. Hansen JP, Drake AL, Walling HW. Bowen's Disease: a four-year retrospective review of epidemiology and treatment at a university center. Dermatol Surg. 2008;34(7):878–83. https://doi.org/10.1111/j.1524-4725.2008.34172.x. PubMed PMID: 18363722.
59. Morton CA, Birnie AJ, Eedy DJ. British Association of Dermatologists' guidelines for the management of squamous cell carcinoma in situ (Bowen's disease) 2014. Br J Dermatol. 2014;170(2):245–60. https://doi.org/10.1111/bjd.12766. PubMed PMID: 24313974.
60. Telfer NR, Colver GB, Morton CA, British Association of Dermatologists. Guidelines for the management of basal cell carcinoma. Br J Dermatol. 2008;159(1):35–48. https://doi.org/10.1111/j.1365-2133.2008.08666.x. PubMed PMID: 18593385.
61. Spiller WF, Spiller RF. Treatment of basal-cell carcinomas by a combination of curettage and cryosurgery. J Dermatol Surg Oncol. 1977;3(4):443–7. PubMed PMID: 893768.
62. Stuart SE, Schoen P, Jin C, Parvataneni R, Arron S, Linos E, et al. Tumor recurrence of keratinocyte carcinomas judged appropriate for Mohs micrographic surgery using Appropriate Use Criteria. J Am Acad Dermatol. 2017;76(6):1131–1138.e1. https://doi.org/10.1016/j.jaad.2016.12.045. PubMed PMID: 28365039; PubMed Central PMCID: PMC5443650.
63. Barlow JO, Zalla MJ, Kyle A, DiCaudo DJ, Lim KK, Yiannias JA. Treatment of basal cell carcinoma with curettage alone. J Am Acad Dermatol. 2006;54(6):1039–45. https://doi.org/10.1016/j.jaad.2006.01.041. PubMed PMID: 16713459.

64. Yakish K, Graham J, Hossler EW. Efficacy of curettage alone for invasive cutaneous squamous cell carcinoma: a retrospective cohort study. J Am Acad Dermatol. 2017;77(3):582–4. https://doi.org/10.1016/j.jaad.2017.04.1108.
65. Jensen NC, Eden A, Robins J, Hull C, Duffy K, Sorensen A, et al. Recurrence rates of keratinocyte carcinoma treated with curettage alone: a retrospective cohort and interview study. Dermatologic Surg. 2022. https://doi.org/10.1097/DSS.0000000000004728.
66. Burkhardt BR, Maw R. Are more passes better? Safety versus efficacy with the pulsed CO2 laser. Plast Reconstr Surg. 1997;100(6):1531–4. PubMed PMID: 9385968.
67. Shaw C. Benign pigmented nevi; a survey of treatment by dermatologists. South Med J. 1953;46(3):286–90. PubMed PMID: 13038544.
68. Walton RG, Cox AJ. Electrodesiccation of pigmented nevi. Arch Dermatol. 1963;87:342–9. https://doi.org/10.1001/archderm.1963.01590150058010. PubMed PMID: 13998746.
69. Slaughter DP. Superficial tumors of the head and neck area. Surg Clin North Am. 1948;28(1):69–81. https://doi.org/10.1016/s0039-6109(16)32332-5. PubMed PMID: 18902059.
70. Walton RG, Sage RD, Farber EM. Electrodesiccation of pigmented nevi; biopsy studies: a preliminary report. AMA Arch Dermatol. 1957;76(2):193–9. https://doi.org/10.1001/archderm.1957.01550200037008. PubMed PMID: 13443505.
71. Tope WD, Sangueza OP. Rhinophyma's fibrous variant. Histopathology and immunohistochemistry. Am J Dermatopathol. 1994;16(3):307–10. PubMed PMID: 7943640.
72. Ambrogi MC, Fanucchi O, Cioni R, Dini P, De LA, Cappelli C, et al. Long-term results of radiofrequency ablation treatment of stage I non-small cell lung cancer: a prospective intention-to-treat study. J Thorac Oncol. 2011;6(1556-1380 (Electronic)):2044–51. https://doi.org/10.1097/JTO.0b013e31822d538d. PubMed PMID: 22052222.
73. Zhang B, Moser M, Zhang E, Zhang WJ. Radiofrequency ablation technique in the treatment of liver tumours: review and future issues. J Med Eng Technol. 2013;37(1464-522X (Electronic)):150–9. https://doi.org/10.3109/03091902.2012.754510. PubMed PMID: 23360198.
74. Taheri A, Mansoori P, Feldman SR, Williford PM, Pearce D. Electrosurgical coagulation of a deep infantile hemangioma using a penetrating insulated electrode: disease modification with minimal superficial scarring. J Am Acad Dermatol. 2013;68(4):AB1, Suplement 1.
75. Braithwaite B, Hnatek L, Zierau U, Camci M, Akkersdijk G, Nio D, et al. Radiofrequency-induced thermal therapy: results of a European multicentre study of resistive ablation of incompetent truncal varicose veins. Phlebology. 2013;28(1758-1125 (Electronic)):38–46. https://doi.org/10.1258/phleb.2012.012013. PubMed PMID: 22865420.
76. Tolva VS, Cireni LV, Bianchi PG, Lombardo A, Keller GC, Casana RM. Radiofrequency ablation of the great saphenous vein with the ClosureFAST procedure: mid-term experience on 400 patients from a single centre. Surg Today. 2012;(1436-2813 (Electronic)). https://doi.org/10.1007/s00595-012-0296-4. PubMed PMID: 22932839.
77. Siribumrungwong B, Noorit P, Wilasrusmee C, Attia J, Thakkinstian A. A systematic review and meta-analysis of randomised controlled trials comparing endovenous ablation and surgical intervention in patients with varicose vein. Eur J Vasc Endovasc Surg. 2012;44(1532-2165 (Electronic)):214–23. https://doi.org/10.1016/j.ejvs.2012.05.017. PubMed PMID: 22705163.
78. Alexiades-Armenakas M, Dover JS, Arndt KA. Unipolar radiofrequency treatment to improve the appearance of cellulite. J Cosmet Laser Ther. 2008;10(1476-4180 (Electronic)):148–53. https://doi.org/10.1080/14764170802279651. PubMed PMID: 18788033.
79. Alexiades-Armenakas M, Dover JS, Arndt KA. Unipolar versus bipolar radiofrequency treatment of rhytides and laxity using a mobile painless delivery method. Lasers Surg Med. 2008;40(1096-9101 (Electronic)):446–53. https://doi.org/10.1002/lsm.20667. PubMed PMID: 18727024.
80. Gold MH, Biron JA. Treatment of acne scars by fractional bipolar radiofrequency energy. J Cosmet Laser Ther. 2012;14(1476-4180 (Electronic)):172–8. https://doi.org/10.3109/14764172.2012.687824. PubMed PMID: 22548644.

81. Brightman L, Goldman MP, Taub AF. Sublative rejuvenation: experience with a new fractional radiofrequency system for skin rejuvenation and repair. J Drugs Dermatol. 2009;8(1545-9616 (Print)):s9–13. PubMed PMID: 19916261.
82. Javate RM, Cruz RT Jr, Khan J, Trakos N, Gordon RE. Nonablative 4-MHz dual radiofrequency wand rejuvenation treatment for periorbital rhytides and midface laxity. Ophthalmic Plast Reconstr Surg. 2011;27(1537-2677 (Electronic)):180–5. https://doi.org/10.1097/IOP.0b013e3181fe8e5a. PubMed PMID: 21283035.
83. Lee SJ, Goo JW, Shin J, Chung WS, Kang JM, Kim YK, et al. Use of fractionated microneedle radiofrequency for the treatment of inflammatory acne vulgaris in 18 Korean patients. Dermatologic Surg. 2012;38(1524-4725 (Electronic)):400–5. https://doi.org/10.1111/j.1524-4725.2011.02267.x. PubMed PMID: 22211476.
84. Sadick NS, Sato M, Palmisano D, Frank I, Cohen H, Harth Y. In vivo animal histology and clinical evaluation of multisource fractional radiofrequency skin resurfacing (FSR) applicator. J Cosmet Laser Ther. 2011;13(1476-4180 (Electronic)):204–9. https://doi.org/10.3109/14764172.2011.606467. PubMed PMID: 21774663.
85. Zelickson BD, Kist D, Bernstein E, Brown DB, Ksenzenko S, Burns J, et al. Histological and ultrastructural evaluation of the effects of a radiofrequency-based nonablative dermal remodeling device: a pilot study. Arch Dermatol. 2004;140(0003-987X (Print)):204–9. https://doi.org/10.1001/archderm.140.2.204. PubMed PMID: 14967794.
86. Krueger N, Sadick NS. New-generation radiofrequency technology. Cutis. 2013;91(0011-4162 (Print)):39–46. PubMed PMID: 23461058.
87. Tan MG, Jo CE, Chapas A, Khetarpal S, Dover JS. Radiofrequency microneedling: a comprehensive and critical review. Dermatologic Surg. 2021;47(6):755. https://doi.org/10.1097/DSS.0000000000002972.
88. Hantash BM, Renton B, Berkowitz RL, Stridde BC, Newman J. Pilot clinical study of a novel minimally invasive bipolar microneedle radiofrequency device. Lasers Surg Med. 2009;41(1096-9101 (Electronic)):87–95. https://doi.org/10.1002/lsm.20687. PubMed PMID: 19226570.
89. Hantash BM, Ubeid AA, Chang H, Kafi R, Renton B. Bipolar fractional radiofrequency treatment induces neoelastogenesis and neocollagenesis. Lasers Surg Med. 2009;41(1096-9101 (Electronic)):1–9. https://doi.org/10.1002/lsm.20731. PubMed PMID: 19143021.
90. Hruza G, Taub AF, Collier SL, Mulholland SR. Skin rejuvenation and wrinkle reduction using a fractional radiofrequency system. J Drugs Dermatol. 2009;8(1545-9616 (Print)):259–65. PubMed PMID: 19271373.
91. Lee HS, Lee DH, Won CH, Chang HW, Kwon HH, Kim KH, et al. Fractional rejuvenation using a novel bipolar radiofrequency system in Asian skin. Dermatologic Surg. 2011;37(1524-4725 (Electronic)):1611–9. https://doi.org/10.1111/j.1524-4725.2011.02134.x. PubMed PMID: 21883650.
92. Seo KY, Yoon MS, Kim DH, Lee HJ. Skin rejuvenation by microneedle fractional radiofrequency treatment in Asian skin; clinical and histological analysis. Lasers Surg Med. 2012;44(1096-9101 (Electronic)):631–6. https://doi.org/10.1002/lsm.22071. PubMed PMID: 22936274.
93. Taheri A, Mansoori P, Sandoval LS, Feldman SR, Williford PM, Pearce D. Entrance and propagation pattern of high-frequency electrical currents in biological tissues as applied to fractional skin rejuvenation using penetrating electrodes. Skin Res Technol. 2014;20(3):270–3.
94. Peterson JD, Palm MD, Kiripolsky MG, Guiha IC, Goldman MP. Evaluation of the effect of fractional laser with radiofrequency and fractionated radiofrequency on the improvement of acne scars. Dermatologic Surg. 2011;37(1524-4725 (Electronic)):1260–7. https://doi.org/10.1111/j.1524-4725.2011.02110.x. PubMed PMID: 21834933.
95. Maness WL, Roeber FW, Clark RE, Cataldo E, Riis D, Haddad AW. Histologic evaluation of electrosurgery with varying frequency and waveform. J Prosthet Dent. 1978;40(0022-3913 (Print)):304–8. PubMed PMID: 279674.

Chapter 6
Electrosurgery and Safety

Abstract An electrosurgical unit is a flexible but complicated surgical tool. Electrosurgery can be associated with some risks to the patients or surgical room staff including burn, electric shock, microorganism transmission, fire, or damage to implanted electronic devices.

6.1 Risks and Potential Complications of Electrosurgery

6.1.1 Neuromuscular Stimulation or Electric Shock

High-frequency alternating electrical currents, such as those used in electrosurgery, do not cause neuromuscular stimulation. However, electrosurgical generators use a low-frequency alternating current as their input power and also have direct current circuits inside their units. These low-frequency or direct currents may leak minimally to the output circuit and may cause minor nerve or muscle stimulation and a feeling of electrical shock. These minor stimulations may cause cardiac arrhythmia if the surgery is done directly on the cardiac muscles during heart surgery. Less commonly, an internal defect in the generator circuits may theoretically cause the low-frequency input power to be connected to the output circuit and cause a major shock to the patient.

There are national and international standards that manufacturers of electrosurgical units should follow to reduce the risk of these potential leakages. Higher-power units and the units used for cardiac surgery should follow more rules and regulations to be approved for use in clinical settings by authorities such as the U.S. Food and Drug Administration.

A. Taheri et al., *Advanced Electrosurgery*,
https://doi.org/10.1007/978-3-032-28342-9_6

6.1.2 Thermoelectric Burns

Electrosurgery is performed by concentrating the current on a small target spot on a surgical site. Unwanted burns on other parts of the patient's body may happen if the current enters or exits the body from a small alternate site. Although this is not a major concern when operating on an alert patient who can sense pain, it can cause major complications in patients who cannot feel or react to pain.

In high-frequency alternating electrical circuits, cables and pathways of electricity always form capacitors with nearby conductive objects. Therefore, high-frequency alternating currents cannot be insulated completely. If the active electrode cable comes in touch with the patient's body, a capacitor is formed that passes some of the current through the insulation on the cable into the patient's body. If electrosurgery is high powered, and the current flow lasts long enough to cause heating of the spot in contact with the cable, an unwanted burn may happen on that spot. Securing the active electrode cable to a surgical drape that is in contact with the patient's body increases this risk, especially if it is done using a metal clamp.

When using an *earth-referenced* electrosurgical unit, the return electrode is connected to the earth (usually through the power cord); therefore, the earth and all conductive objects around the patient's body act as a capacitive-type dispersive electrode. Earth-referenced units can be operated in monoterminal or single-electrode mode with no return electrode connected to the patient's body. During monoterminal electrosurgery (no return electrode connected), if an electrically conductive object, such as a metal table, electrocardiogram electrode, or surgical staff, comes into contact with the patient's body, some current may select that object as a low resistance return pathway to the ground. If the contact area is small, the current concentration at this point may result in a burn. To reduce this risk, the monoterminal mode is used only on conscious patients who can feel pain and only on insulated surgical tables. Using a return electrode reduces the risk of this type of burn by ensuring that the current returns to the device through the path of least resistance and not taking any alternative path through environmental objects.

Although a good dispersive electrode reduces the risk of distant site burns, inadequate contact of the dispersive electrode with the patient's body may result in a smaller contact area that can concentrate the current and cause a burn. Some electrosurgical units have a contact quality monitor for the dispersive electrode, which measures the quality of the contact between the patient's skin and the dispersive electrode and also between the electrode and the generator. Contact quality is monitored by splitting the return electrode into two parts and measuring the electrical resistance between the parts. If one or both parts are not in good contact with the skin or the device, the resistance in the return electrode circuit will be high, and the monitoring system will disable the generator.

The best location for placement of the dispersive electrode is a muscular or flat site, well supplied with blood vessels and adjacent to the surgical field. If there is any metal or implanted electronic device in the patient's body, it should not be placed between the active and dispersive electrodes or close to them. When performing high-power electrosurgery on an unconscious patient, the return electrode should not be placed under the patient's body at pressure points such as under the buttocks, heel, or upper back. The weight of the patient may cause enough pressure on those spots to slow down or stop blood circulation. With slow blood circulation under the return electrode, there is a greater risk of an increase in temperature to the levels that may cause a burn.

Performing a high-power monopolar electrosurgery on an extremity such as a finger or penis may result in heating and burning of the whole extremity. When applying an electrosurgical current to a fingertip, there is a limited cross-sectional area for the return current to spread across. Theoretically, this may result in higher current density and some heating throughout the volume of the extremity. In order to avoid this complication, a very-low-power current can be used, or the activation time can be short. Wrapping the target finger to adjacent fingers using gauze soaked in saline can help increase the cross-sectional area for the return current to spread across. Achieving a deep electrocoagulation on a relatively large surface area needs a lot of energy and heat production and is generally not recommended, especially on a finger, where a deep coagulation will reach bones.

6.1.3 Damage to the Anatomic Structures Underneath the Target

One of the limitations of electrosurgery is that the depth of coagulation is not visible during the procedure. A deep coagulation of the skin may extend to subcutaneous tissue and affect the underlying nerves, arteries, cartilages, or bones. Injecting saline or lidocaine into the superficial subcutaneous plane under the target can elevate the skin and isolate it from the deeper tissues, reducing the risk of damage to underlying structures during the procedure.

6.1.4 Microorganism Transmission

Any electrosurgical procedure that involves spark formation can cause high enough temperatures for charring tissue and smoke formation. Smoke from electrosection or electrofulguration can contain toxic gases and vapors such as benzene, hydrogen cyanide, and formaldehyde. While some animal studies show that very high concentrations of these gases can cause pulmonary or eye problems, there is no strong evidence that a routine electrosurgical procedure in an average surgical room can cause a high smoke concentration in the air higher than the levels in our kitchens, restaurants, around our grills, or in streets in larger cities with air pollution.

Smoke from thermal charring of tissue should not have any viable organisms, thanks to the sterilization effect of high temperature needed for charring and smoke formation. However, tissue explosion or explosion of bubbles that form from boiling water may send some tissue or blood particles into the air. There is some concern that some of those particles may never reach a temperature high enough for sterilization and may have viable organisms or cells. This possibility has not been investigated thoroughly in clinical settings.

Papillomavirus DNA and human immunodeficiency virus DNA have been found using polymerase chain reaction (PCR) or other amplification techniques in the vapor (smoke plume) derived from infected tissue treated with electrosurgery or ablative lasers. One should bear in mind that PCR can detect DNA particles of the viruses that have been killed by heat, and so it does not prove the infectivity or viability of the germs in the specimen. There is one report of clinical infection with bovine papillomavirus infection when the laser plume (aerosol) from infected cells was suctioned and collected and then reinoculated onto the skin of calves [1]. Other studies failed to find any virulent or viable virus or tumoral cells in electrosurgical smoke. There has also not been any report of viral transmission associated with surgical smoke in clinical settings [2–6].

Portable surgical smoke evacuators can effectively control potential airborne contaminants generated by electrosurgery as well as unpleasant odors. However, most dermatologic surgeons do not use those systems unless the tissue treated is known to have viruses such as HIV or HPV. One large survey study found that only 10% of dermatologic surgeons utilize smoke management practices [7]. Surgical masks such as N-95 or respirators are other alternatives but probably inferior to the evacuators. The effectiveness of those measures has not been studied in clinical settings.

Microorganism transmission is also possible through active electrodes. The surgeons can minimize this risk by using disposable or sterilized electrodes. Adapters, such as electrolysis electrodes that hold electrolysis needles, are available that allow disposable metal hypodermic needles to be used as electrodes. The surgeons may break the plastic end of hypodermic needles and use the metal part as a low-cost disposable electrode.

6.1.5 Fire

Sparks formed during electrosurgery may cause fire or explosion if electrosurgery is conducted in the presence of flammable materials such as alcohol, bowel gases (methane), or a very high concentration of oxygen.

Care should be taken to be certain that the operative site is free of alcohol residue.

Oxygen itself is not flammable in the absence of any fuel. However, other flammable materials, such as dry surgical gauze or drapes, burn faster and may explode in the presence of a high concentration of oxygen. If electrosurgery is performed on the face in the presence of nasal oxygen, oxygen may need to be stopped a few seconds before electrosurgery. We should bear in mind that porous flammable material, such as gauze, can keep oxygen inside for a few seconds. Making surgical gauze damp reduces the risk of fire in the presence of high concentrations of oxygen.

Bowel gases may include methane and may be flammable. This is a concern mainly during electrosurgery on the bowels. There has not been any report of fire associated with bowel gases during electrosurgery on perianal skin.

6.2 Electrosurgery and Implantable Electronic Devices

Electronic devices implanted in patients' bodies may be affected by external electromagnetic fields or electrical currents. A strong electrosurgical current passing through an electronic device may cause permanent damage to the device, alter its programming, or interfere with its function transiently. Recent improvements in electrical shielding and filtering systems have made implanted electronic devices more resistant to outside electrical interference [8]. While very powerful electromagnetic fields or currents (e.g., a high-power monopolar electrosurgery very close to the device or its leads) may have permanent effects on a device, relatively weaker electromagnetic fields or currents may only interfere transiently with device function, and when the interference ceases, the device returns to its normal function.

The incidence of interference is higher when using monopolar rather than bipolar electrosurgery, using a higher power, working near the implanted device, or having the device between the active and dispersive electrode [9].

There is limited clinical trial data available to guide surgeons on how to use electrosurgery on patients with implanted electronic devices. Therefore, most guidelines published by experts or medical societies are based on case reports, retrospective studies, laboratory research, or manufacturers' recommendations. Recommendations offered in this chapter are mainly based on the British Society for Dermatological Surgery and British Heart Rhythm Society Guidance, revised 2023 [10].

Although implanted electronic devices are used in multiple organs for neuromuscular stimulation or recording, electromagnetic interference is a major concern only when electrosurgery causes inhibition of cardiac pacemakers or inappropriate activation of implantable cardioverter defibrillators (ICDs). Transient electromagnetic interference with other implanted devices is usually of no major concern.

6.2.1 Cardiac Implantable Electronic Devices

Cardiac implantable electronic devices are used as pacemakers for the treatment of bradycardia or heart block, resynchronization pacemakers for the management of heart failure, ICDs for the treatment of life-threatening ventricular tachycardias, implantable heart failure monitoring systems, or implantable loop recorders and insertable cardiac monitors for monitoring cardiac rhythm.

Implanted Cardiac Monitors

Implantable loop recorders and insertable cardiac monitors have been made only to monitor cardiac signals. The device may interpret electromagnetic interference as a rapid heart rhythm and record an episode of tachycardia, but this will be apparent when the device is interrogated. High-power electrosurgery very close to the device may cause damage to the recorder; otherwise, electrosurgery has no risk to the patient, and therefore no additional precautions are needed during surgery for patients with implantable loop recorders or insertable cardiac monitors. Before any monopolar electrosurgery close to the device, the cardiology team should be informed that a procedure is planned, to give them the opportunity to download the stored data from the recorder beforehand.

Implantable Heart Failure Monitoring Systems

Implantable heart failure monitoring devices estimate intravascular fluid status of patients by sensing pulmonary artery, atrial, or vena cava pressure. The data is transmitted to the cardiology team to be used for better management of heart failure. The cardiology team can monitor the patients remotely and call or visit them if the data shows that the patient is volume overloaded.

Electrosurgery or any other electromagnetic interference may temporarily affect implanted heart failure monitoring sensor readings but does not generally damage the implant.

6.2.1.1 Cardiac Pacemakers

A cardiac pacemaker initiates pacing for the heart if the heart does not produce enough electrical activity or if the signals do not travel to the ventricles appropriately. Some hearts that are supported by pacemakers may produce enough electrical activity most of the time and may not be dependent on the pacemaker at the time of surgery. If a pacemaker is programmed as on-demand, it does not pace if it detects enough cardiac electrical activity. Electrosurgery on a patient with a heart that is not dependent on a pacemaker at the time of surgery may not cause any problem. However, in a pace-dependent patient, the pacemaker may misinterpret electrosurgical currents as cardiac activity and may stop pacing. This may result in bradycardia or asystole if electrosurgical currents are applied for a prolonged period of time. This risk is higher if the procedure is high power and is in proximity to the device. If bradycardia or asystole happens, stopping the electrosurgical current will result in reactivation of the pacemaker. Then, short bursts of electrosurgery can be used with enough time between the bursts for the pacemaker to run the heart. If this is not feasible, reprogramming the device to a fixed-rate pacing mode (also called asynchronous mode or not on-demand) should be considered. Alternatively, a magnet can be placed on the pulse generator site to change the behavior to an asynchronous pacing.

Determining Pacing Dependency

The presence of pacing stimulation artifacts on an ECG means that the pacemaker runs the heart, but it does not mean that the person is pacemaker-dependent. Pacemaker dependency is usually defined as hemodynamic instability with the intrinsic rhythm or no intrinsic rhythm >40 beats per minute. Most patients with a pacemaker are not pacemaker-dependent based on this definition, and, as such, if their device is temporarily turned off, it would not cause any problem.

Pacing Modes

Understanding pacing modes helps with a more in-depth understanding of the potential effects of electrosurgical currents on pacemaker function (Table 6.1).

In response to a sensed intracardiac signal, a pacemaker may inhibit its output, trigger an output, or pace in a different chamber. This function is governed by the programmed pacing mode. The pacing mode of a pacemaker can be reprogrammed based on the patient's needs and heart status.

Reprogramming of pacemakers before or after surgery can be performed by a technician using an external device that communicates with the pacemaker. Another way to change the programming of a pacemaker is to place a magnet over the pulse generator site. Most pacemakers respond with fixed-rate (asynchronous) pacing while a magnet is held over the generator. While this can be useful in rare situations where pacing is inhibited by electrosurgical currents, leaving a magnet over the pacemaker is not generally needed or recommended. The asynchronous pacing can be arrhythmogenic very rarely in patients with an underlying intrinsic cardiac rhythm (R-on-T phenomenon).

Pacemakers that are parts of ICDs and some leadless pacemakers may not have any response to magnets.

Table 6.1 Common pacing modes, their clinical applications, and effect of electromagnetic fields on them

Pacing mode	Clinical application	Effect of external electromagnetic fields on the pacemaker function
Single-chamber atrial pacemaker	Isolated sinus node dysfunction with intact AV nodal conduction. If the intrinsic sinus rate drops below the programmed rate, pacing occurs	The pacemaker may sense the electrosurgical current and misinterpret it as normal cardiac activity and pause pacing. In case there is not enough true cardiac activity, and the heart is pace-dependent, this pause in pace causes bradycardia or asystole as long as the interference exists
Ventricular-only pacing	Patients with chronic atrial fibrillation, or infrequent pauses or bradycardias. The potential for tracking atrial arrhythmias is eliminated. If the ventricular rate drops below the programmed rate, pacing occurs	The pacemaker may sense the electrosurgical current and misinterpret it as normal cardiac activity and pause pacing. In case there is not enough true cardiac activity, and the heart is pace-dependent, this pause in pace causes bradycardia or asystole as long as the interference exists

(continued)

Table 6.1 (continued)

Pacing mode	Clinical application	Effect of external electromagnetic fields on the pacemaker function
Standard dual-chamber pacing. This is the most commonly used pacemaker mode	AV nodal conduction disease or sinus node dysfunction. The device will sense and pace in both atrium and ventricle based on the sinus rate, physiologic demand, or AV conduction at each moment	The pacemaker may sense the electrosurgical current and misinterpret it as normal cardiac activity and pause pacing The pacemaker may sense the electrosurgical current and misinterpret it as normal atrial activity, track it, and pace inappropriately in the ventricle. This is unlikely to lead to any clinical harm
Asynchronous or fixed-rate modes	Asynchronous pacing delivers electrical stimuli at a programmed rate, regardless of the heart's intrinsic electrical activity. These modes prevent sensing of extrinsic electrical activity, which may be "misinterpreted" as native cardiac events, inhibiting pacing, or leading to rapid ventricular pacing. This mode is usually a temporary mode programmed to avoid recognition of external electromagnetic activities, including electrosurgery	No effect on pacemaker function
Rate response (also called rate-adaptive pacing)	This mode enables the pacemaker to increase the pacing rate in response to physical, mental, or emotional exertion. Different physiological sensors have been used to predict the need for a higher heart rate. One of these sensors is the Minute Ventilation Sensor which senses pulmonary impedance that occurs with respiration and increases the heart rate if the respiratory rate increases	It may cause sensor error and increase the heart rate, similar to what happens during exercise. This is unlikely to lead to any clinical harm

6.2.1.2 Implantable Cardioverter Defibrillators (ICDs)

ICDs are implanted in patients who are considered high risk or have a history of fatal ventricular arrhythmias. An ICD delivers a shock to treat those arrhythmias if the device detects them; hence, there is the possibility that electromagnetic interference may be misinterpreted as ventricular arrhythmia, causing inappropriate delivery of shocks.

Most of the patients with ICD do not have an indication for a permanent pacemaker, and their device may be programmed to pace the heart only if the heart rate is <40 beats per minute. Some of the ICDs have a special pacemaker mode called cardiac resynchronization therapy. These devices are implanted to treat patients with heart failure who also have underlying significant interventricular conduction delays or blocks. These devices work by reorganizing an appropriate flow of electrical activities in the heart. In most of these patients, a transient pause in resynchronization therapy does not cause any major hemodynamic changes and does not cause any harm.

Manufacturers of implantable ICDs either contraindicate the use of electrosurgery or give strong warnings against its use, especially with the monopolar mode of operation. However, electrosurgery at a site remote from the implanted device has a relatively low risk of interference that may lead to inappropriate delivery of shocks. The use of bipolar electrosurgery reduces, but does not eliminate, this risk.

Pre- and Intraoperative Management of Patients with a Pacemaker or ICD
There is limited clinical trial data or evidence-based recommendations available to guide us on how to use electrosurgery on patients with a pacemaker or ICD. Recommendations offered here are mainly based on the British Society for Dermatological Surgery and British Heart Rhythm Society Guidance revised 2023 (Table 6.2) and the American Heart Association statement 2024 [10, 11].

The American Heart Association has recommendations similar to British Heart Rhythm Society. They recommend disabling ICDs if surgical site is above umbilicus (recommendations are different if pacemaker is in abdomen). Disabling ICD can be done using a magnet or reprograming the device, depending on pacing dependency, patient positioning, or recommendations from the CIED team [11].

The American Heart Association suggests considering asynchronous pacing mode for pacing-dependent patients if surgical site is above umbilicus [11].

The following care should be considered when electrosurgery is used on patients with a cardiac pacemaker or ICD:

- Use the minimum power settings required for adequate electrosurgery and consider the bipolar mode. For monopolar electrosurgery, place the return electrode at a site where the current path is kept as far as possible from the implanted electronic device.
- Using short bursts of electrosurgery (bursts less than 5 second durations with rest periods between the bursts) is less likely to cause problems associated with pacemaker inhibition. However, in patients with ICDs, even short bursts of electrosurgery might be interpreted as native ventricular arrhythmia and lead to inappropriate shocks. Hence, the recommendation is to disable the tachyarrhythmia detections in ICD patients, especially when the site is above the umbilicus.
- Monitoring the patient's ECG from the outset of the procedure is preferable (some monitors may give inaccurate readings of paced beats, so if in doubt, check the patient's pulse and/or use pulse oximetry). If the patient is awake and it is possible to maintain verbal contact during the procedure, then pulse oximetry monitoring alone is an acceptable alternative to ECG monitoring.

Table 6.2 British Heart Rhythm Society guideline on pre- and intraoperative management of patients with pacemakers or ICDs who may need electrosurgery [10]

	Pacemaker		ICD	
Surgery site	Pacing-dependent	Not pacing-dependent	Pacing-dependent	Not pacing-dependent
Surgery above umbilicus	Consider reprogramming to a fixed rate if prolonged electrosurgery is anticipated[a]	Monitor during surgery to ensure no inhibition of pacemaker. No reprogramming	Deactivate ICD[b] and consider reprogramming to fixed-rate pacing or magnet application as an alternative only if prolonged electrosurgery is not anticipated	Deactivate ICD[b] or magnet application
Surgery below umbilicus	Monitor during surgery to ensure no inhibition of pacemaker. No reprogramming. Clinical magnets should be available	Monitor during surgery to ensure no inhibition of pacemaker. No reprogramming	Monitor during surgery to ensure no inhibition of pacemaker or inappropriate ICD activation. Reasonable not to deactivate ICD. Clinical magnet should be available	

[a]For dermatological surgery, pacemaker reprogramming needs only to be considered if the patient is pacemaker-dependent, if long bursts of electrosurgery more than 5 seconds are needed, and the surgical site is within 5 cm of the device

[b]Suspension of ICD treatment can be achieved by either (1) deactivation of the device by a member of the cardiac team using a programmer or (2) by temporary application of a clinical magnet. There are practical advantages and disadvantages to these approaches. Deactivation is a more definite approach; however, it requires input from the cardiac team before and after surgery (which can be challenging logistically), and while the device is awaiting reactivation, it will not treat potentially serious arrhythmias. Magnet deactivation is an alternative where cardiac physiologists are not on-site, and it reduces the risk that patients fail to have therapies turned on after surgery. A potential disadvantage of magnet deactivation is that the magnet may be positioned inappropriately or move unintentionally away from the device

ICD implantable cardioverter defibrillator

- External defibrillation and cardiopulmonary resuscitation equipment should be readily available, ideally with external temporary pacing capacity.
- If electrosurgery is an essential and unavoidable part of the planned surgery, a clinical magnet should be available for any patient who has an ICD where reprogramming has not been undertaken.

Although highly unlikely, if pacemaker interference (bradycardia or inappropriate rapid pacing) occurs during electrosurgery, prompt cessation thereof will resume normal device function. If further electrosurgery is required, shorter bursts may be attempted. If continued and symptomatic interference occurs, magnet application or device reprogramming may be carried out. If electrosurgery triggers an ICD shock and further electrosurgery is required, magnet application or device reprogramming will stop ICD from shocking.

Table 6.3 Parameters that determine the risk of electrosurgery on patients with pacemaker or ICD

Low risk	Medium risk	High risk
Pacemaker		ICD
Pacemaker-nondependent	Pacemaker-dependent	
Electrosurgery below umbilicus	Electrosurgery above umbilicus	Electrosurgery within 5 cm of device
Bipolar electrosurgery		Monopolar electrosurgery
Low-power electrosurgery		High-power electrosurgery

ICD implantable cardioverter defibrillator

The British Heart Rhythm Society recommends preoperative cardiology or cardiac electrophysiology team consultation for all patients with ICD who need electrosurgery and for patients with a pacemaker within 5 cm of the electrosurgical site. However, because of very low rates of reported complications, some dermatologists may consult cardiology only before the highest risk surgeries, including monopolar electrosurgery above the umbilicus on patients with ICD (Table 6.3).

Magnet Use on a Pacemaker or ICD

Pacemakers or ICDs respond to the placement of a magnet over them in a variety of ways. The response to the presence of a magnet in both pacemakers and ICDs is only temporary, and normal function will resume as soon as the magnet is removed.

Clinical magnets for this application will be available from cardiology centers along with instructions for correct use.

Pacemaker Magnet Response

Most pacemakers (simple and resynchronization) respond with a fixed rate (asynchronous) pacing while a magnet is held over the generator.

Leadless pacemakers may not have any response to magnets.

ICD Magnet Response

For ICDs, placing a magnet over the device will inhibit the delivery of anti-tachycardia pacing and shock therapy but will not affect bradycardia pacing.

6.2.2 Neuromodulation Implantable Electronic Devices

In neuromodulation, an implanted electronic device, also called neurostimulator, is used to modulate neural activity in the central or peripheral nervous system. A typical neurostimulator has an implantable pulse generator (IPG) and one or more electrode(s) that deliver electrical impulses to the target. Insulated extension cables, tunneled subcutaneously, connect the IPG with the electrodes (Fig. 6.1).

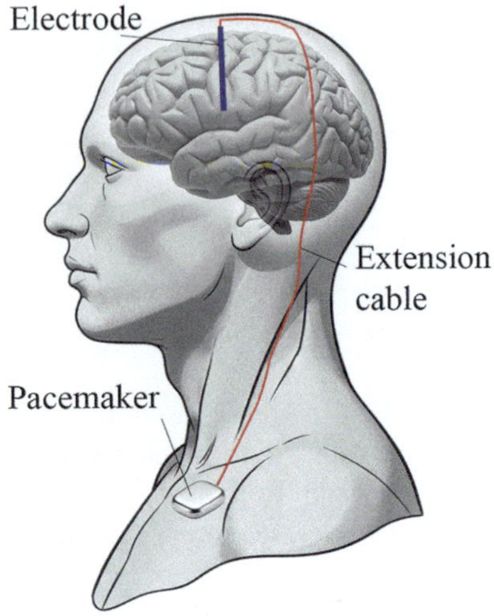

Fig. 6.1 A typical implanted deep brain stimulator

After surgical implantation, the device is turned on and "programmed." This means that the parameters are adjusted to obtain the best symptom control while avoiding stimulation-related adverse effects (discussed below) and optimizing battery efficiency. Such parameters typically include voltage, current intensity, pulse width, pulse frequency, and stimulation mode.

For programming, the clinician uses an external programmer device to communicate with IPG wirelessly. The patient is also given a controller device which allows for limited changes, including turning the device on/off or small changes in a couple of parameters.

Neurostimulators in clinical use include:

- Spinal cord stimulation (SCS): This is the first and most common neurostimulator used in modern clinical practice. It is typically used to treat chronic intractable (usually neuropathic) pain in back or lower extremities such as in failed back surgery syndrome. In SCS, an electrode is placed in the epidural space of the spinal cord and is connected to the IPG buried in the subcutaneous tissue of the lower back, upper gluteal, or abdominal region, via insulated leads tunneled subcutaneously.
- Deep brain stimulation (DBS): This modality is the second most common clinically used neurostimulator. The most common approved indication for DBS is Parkinson's disease, but it can be used in treatment of several other ailments, and the list is growing: essential tremor, dystonia, epilepsy, psychiatric conditions, obesity, and addiction. The target of stimulation in the brain varies depending on the disease to be treated. For example, in Parkinson's disease, the electrode is usually inserted in the subthalamic nucleus or globus pallidus. The IPG is usually implanted in subclavicular region.

- Sacral nerve stimulation (SNS): The electrode is inserted through the sacral foramina (usually S3 or S4) and is connected to the IPG in the upper gluteal region. The most common indication for SNS is certain kinds of urinary incontinence.
- Vagus nerve stimulation (VNS): The electrode is wrapped around the left vagus nerve in the carotid sheath (in the neck) and connected to the IPG in the subclavicular region. VNS is considered in the treatment of resistant epilepsy or depression.
- Cochlear implants are used to treat severe sensorineural hearing loss. It is inserted through an incision in the mastoid region.
- Various forms of peripheral nerve stimulators used for chronic neuropathic pain.
- Dorsal root ganglion (DRG) stimulation which blocks or modulates pain signals traveling from periphery toward CNS centers.
- Phrenic nerve stimulation (also called diaphragmatic pacing) is used in the treatment of respiratory insufficiency due to high cervical spinal cord injury, diaphragmatic paralysis, or central sleep apnea.
- Hypoglossal nerve stimulation, an innovative therapy used to treat obstructive sleep apnea.
- Gastric electrical stimulator used for the treatment of gastroparesis.

SCS works mainly by blocking spine pathways of pain. The "gate control theory" of pain signal transmission at spinal level is thought to be involved. Gate control theory also plays a role in peripheral nerve and DRG stimulation to treat pain although other mechanisms have also been proposed.

In the case of DBS, there are several hypotheses describing the phenomenon from a particular perspective and at various scales. The neurophysiological effects of DBS include local and network-wide suppression and/or activation, neurochemical effects, modulation of oscillatory activity, and synaptic plasticity.

Apart from general surgical complications such as infection or wound problems, complications of neuromodulation can be related to device malfunction/failure or stimulation-related issues.

Stimulation-related adverse effects include paresthesia or tingling sensation, visual changes, speech or motor changes, mood disturbance, autonomic dysregulation, etc. Those adverse effects can result from either overstimulation of the intended target or electrical stimulation of other neural structures adjacent to the planned target. For instance, in stimulation of subthalamic nucleus, current spread to adjacent optic tract can cause various visual adverse effects including phosphene (perception of light), blurring of vision, or visual field defects. Another common example is tingling sensation or muscle twitching in lower extremities as a consequence of overstimulation in SCS.

Potential Adverse Effects of Electrosurgery on Neuromodulation Device

Electrosurgery can damage the device or interfere with neurostimulator function in several ways:

- Direct thermal or mechanical damage to the IPG, electrode, or the extension lead.

- Sending the electrosurgical current down the electrode. In this case, the electrode acts as an extension of the electrosurgery probe and can cause tissue damage at the site of electrode contacts. For example, in a DBS system, it can cause thermal damage at the deep target within the brain parenchyma.
- Temporary suppression or inappropriate activation of the neurostimulator.
- Changing the device setting and its parameters, hence causing device malfunction.

Abrupt discontinuation or erratic reprogramming of the neurostimulator can happen during the use of electrosurgery. The obvious expected consequence of device deactivation is symptom rebound such as rigidity, freezing, and tremor in Parkinson's disease or pain in a patient harboring SCS. Note that the medication dosage is usually reduced after the administration of neuromodulation; thus, the patient is dependent on neurostimulation for adequate symptom control. Sometimes these rebound symptoms can be even more severe than their original baseline due to central sensitization. Other consequences include autonomic dysregulation and psychological changes.

Erratic parameter changes can lead to either overstimulation or underdelivery of neuromodulation therapy and inadequate symptom control.

Safety Measures for Electrosurgery in a Patient with an Implanted Neuromodulation Electronic Device

There is limited clinical data available to guide us on how to manage the patients with a neurostimulator who need electrosurgery. Therefore, most recommendations are based on case reports or series, manufacturers' recommendations, and our experience with cardiac pacemakers which are analogous to neurostimulators.

Similar to cardiac pacemakers, electrosurgery is generally safe if the treatment team takes safety precautions especially when working far from the neurostimulator [12, 13]. When the risk of device-related problems is deemed significant (e.g., a lengthy, high-power, monopolar electrosurgery near the neurostimulator), the device manufacturer and/or the physician in charge of neuromodulation can be contacted for further help.

In addition to general recommendations for performing electrosurgery in the presence of an implanted electronic device (discussed earlier in this chapter), the following recommendations also apply in patients having any form of implanted device in the nervous system:

- Bipolar electrosurgery is generally safer than monopolar in the presence of implanted electronic devices.
- Locate the neurostimulator components before the surgery. This may necessitate taking an X-ray of the relevant body parts, especially if the surgical field is near the device.
- Stay away from the neurostimulator components by a margin of at least 3 cm, even when using a bipolar electrode.
- Use the lowest possible power setting (current and voltage) for electrosurgery.

- When using monopolar electrosurgery, the dispersive electrode should be placed in a location to direct the electric currents away from the neurostimulator.
- If performing high-power monopolar electrosurgery near the neurostimulator is inevitable, use intermittent, short bursts to reduce the risk of thermal damage to the device that may happen if the current passes through the neurostimulator circuits.
- Some Abbott's DBS systems have a dedicated "surgery mode." In most other neurostimulators, it is advised to turn the device off before electrosurgery to minimize the risk of device malfunction or damage and prevent electromagnetic interference with other electronic instruments in the operating room such as ECG monitoring. The device can be turned off before surgery to check if the patient can tolerate the discontinuation of stimulation.
- Before turning off the neurostimulator, set its parameters such as voltage and amplitude to the lowest power possible so that in case the device inadvertently turns on during the electrosurgery (due to electromagnetic interference), the risks such as overstimulation are minimized.
- Always disconnect any external stimulation before electrosurgery. External stimulation is commonly used in the trial phase of SCS and SNS before connecting the electrode to the IPG for permanent neurostimulation.
- During the pre-op preparations, consider adjusting the patient's medications so that the disruption of neurostimulation causes minimal discomfort to the patient. This may require consulting the relevant clinician.

References

1. Garden JM, O'Banion MK, Bakus AD, Olson C. Viral disease transmitted by laser-generated plume (aerosol). Arch Dermatol. 2002;138(10):1303–7. https://doi.org/10.1001/archderm.138.10.1303.
2. Baggish MS, Poiesz BJ, Joret D, Williamson P, Refai A. Presence of human immunodeficiency virus DNA in laser smoke. Lasers Surg Med. 1991;11(3):197–203. https://doi.org/10.1002/lsm.1900110302.
3. Sawchuk WS, Weber PJ, Lowy DR, Dzubow LM. Infectious papillomavirus in the vapor of warts treated with carbon dioxide laser or electrocoagulation: detection and protection. J Am Acad Dermatol. 1989;21(1):41–9. https://doi.org/10.1016/s0190-9622(89)70146-8.
4. Georgesen C, Lipner SR. Surgical smoke: risk assessment and mitigation strategies. J Am Acad Dermatol. 2018;79(4):746–55. https://doi.org/10.1016/j.jaad.2018.06.003.
5. Lewin JM, Brauer JA, Ostad A. Surgical smoke and the dermatologist. J Am Acad Dermatol. 2011;65(3):636–41. https://doi.org/10.1016/j.jaad.2010.11.017.
6. Oosterhuis JW, Verschueren RC, Eibergen R, Oldhoff J. The viability of cells in the waste products of CO2-laser evaporation of Cloudman mouse melanomas. Cancer. 1982;49(1):61–7. https://doi.org/10.1002/1097-0142(19820101)49:1<61::aid-cncr2820490114>3.0.co;2-n.
7. Oganesyan G, Eimpunth S, Kim SS, Jiang SIB. Surgical smoke in dermatologic surgery. Dermatol Surg. 2014;40(12):1373–7. https://doi.org/10.1097/DSS.0000000000000221.
8. Voutsalath MA, Bichakjian CK, Pelosi F, Blum D, Johnson TM, Farrehi PM. Electrosurgery and implantable electronic devices: review and implications for office-based procedures. Dermatol Surg. 2011;37(1524–4725 (Electronic)):889–99. https://doi.org/10.1111/j.1524-4725.2011.02006.x.

9. Govekar HR, Robinson TN, Varosy PD, Girard G, Montero PN, Dunn CL, et al. Effect of monopolar radiofrequency energy on pacemaker function. Surg Endosc. 2012;26(1432–2218 (Electronic)):2784–8. https://doi.org/10.1007/s00464-012-2279-3.
10. BHRS guidelines - management of patients with Cardiac Implantable Electronic Devices (CIEDs) around the time of surgery. British Heart Rhythm Society [Internet]. [cited 2025 Jul 29]. Available from: https://bhrs.com/document/bhrs-guidelines-managment-of-patients-with-cardiac-implantable-electronic-devices-cieds-around-the-time-of-surgery-revised-oct-2023/.
11. Wan EY, Rogers AJ, Lavelle M, Marcus M, Stone SA, Ottoboni L, et al. Periprocedural management and multidisciplinary care pathways for patients with cardiac implantable electronic devices: a scientific statement from the American Heart Association. Circulation. 2024;150(8):e183–96. https://doi.org/10.1161/CIR.0000000000001264.
12. McMahon R, Morgan SJ, Brooks JT, Cahill P, Fitzgerald R, Li Y, et al. Does the presence of programmable implanted devices in patients with early onset scoliosis alter typical operative and postoperative practices? A survey of spine surgeons. Spine Deform. 2022;10(4):951–64. https://doi.org/10.1007/s43390-022-00477-w.
13. Abdul-Rahman NH, Choi AY, Ravuri S, Whelan RL, Soose RJ, Kaffenberger TM. Safety of monopolar electrocautery use in patients with implanted hypoglossal nerve stimulators. Laryngoscope. 2025;135(11):4442–8. https://doi.org/10.1002/lary.32291.

Appendix

International Electrotechnical Committee (IEC) Symbols for Safety Level of Electromedical Devices

Of note, these standards are used by medical engineers for categorizing electrosurgical devices. These recommendations are usually based on in vitro studies and tests.

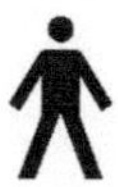 Type B Applied Part: Complying with specified requirements for earth reference devices for protection against electric shock. This is the basic level of safety used mainly in earth-referenced electrosurgical devices. These devices are usually low power or are used in an outpatient setting on alert patients who can report an electrical burn on an area other than the surgical site.

 Type BF Applied Part: A floated (isolated from earth, not earth-referenced) device complying with specified requirements for floated devices for protection against electric shock. Type BF has a higher degree of protection against electric shock than type B applied parts. The chance of burn is less for patients and also for the surgical room staff. Most of the high-power modern electrosurgical units are this type.

 Type CF Applied Part: A floated (isolated from earth, not earth-referenced) device complying with specified requirements for floated devices for protection against electric shock during cardiac surgery. Type CF has the highest degree of

A. Taheri et al., *Advanced Electrosurgery*,
https://doi.org/10.1007/978-3-032-28342-9

protection against electric shock, higher than type BF and type B applied parts. This is the only type that can come in direct contact with the heart during heart surgery.

 Defibrillation-Proof Devices: These devices are protected against damage caused by electrical shocks produced by a defibrillator.

Index

A. Taheri et al., *Advanced Electrosurgery*,
https://doi.org/10.1007/978-3-032-28342-9

MIX
Papier aus verantwortungsvollen Quellen
Paper from responsible sources
FSC® C105338

If you have any concerns about our products,
you can contact us on
ProductSafety@springernature.com

In case Publisher is established outside the EU,
the EU authorized representative is:
Springer Nature Customer Service Center GmbH
Europaplatz 3, 69115 Heidelberg, Germany

Printed by Libri Plureos GmbH
in Hamburg, Germany